PRAISE FOR

happy herbivore light & lean

"Lindsay Nixon knocks it out of the park with *Happy Herbivore Light & Lean*. Eat these delicious recipes, start engaging in these low-impact exercises, and watch a health kingdom emerge from within."

—RIP ESSELSTYN, *NEW YORK TIMES* BESTSELLING AUTHOR OF *MY BEEF WITH MEAT*

"Lindsay Nixon now is a household name in developing cookbooks that have the kind of recipes for the future that are healthful, tasty, and easy to prepare. Here's another that you need for your collection."

—T. COLIN CAMPBELL, COAUTHOR OF *THE CHINA STUDY* AND THE *NEW YORK TIMES* BESTSELLING *WHOLE*, AND KAREN CAMPBELL

"No comment can truly capture the totality of Lindsay's magic in the kitchen! Once again, in *Happy Herbivore Light & Lean*, she creatively proves that plant-based eating is not only delicious but also low-calorie and so satisfying."

—CALDWELL B. ESSELSTYN, JR., MD, AUTHOR OF *PREVENT AND REVERSE HEART DISEASE*, AND ANN CRILE ESSELSTYN

"*Happy Herbivore Light & Lean* is a wonderful book full of simple, delicious meals to get you started on a healthy vegan diet. Lindsay not only provides a wealth of creative plant-based recipes but also gives great tips to help you lose weight, gain energy, and feel fantastic. I invite everyone to read this excellent new book and get started on your journey to health."

—NEAL BARNARD, MD, FOUNDER AND PRESIDENT OF THE PHYSICIANS COMMITTEE FOR RESPONSIBLE MEDICINE

"Lindsay Nixon has done it again! Another fantastic cookbook filled with easy, delicious, low-fat vegan recipes that everyone will love. Recommended to all McDougall Program followers as well as anyone desiring better health through healthy eating."

—JOHN AND MARY MCDOUGALL, BESTSELLING AUTHORS AND FOUNDERS OF THE MCDOUGALL PROGRAM

"I am thrilled to discover in her new cookbook what many of you have known for a while—that girl can cook!"

—DEL SROUFE, AUTHOR OF *BETTER THAN VEGAN* AND *FORKS OVER KNIVES—THE COOKBOOK*

"*Happy Herbivore Light & Lean* provides inventive, easy-to-make recipes and sensible do-it-yourself exercises, to get you on the road to excellent health."

—BRIAN WENDEL, EXECUTIVE PRODUCER, *FORKS OVER KNIVES*

More Cookbooks in Lindsay S. Nixon's

Happy Herbivore Series

The Happy Herbivore Cookbook

Everyday Happy Herbivore

Happy Herbivore Abroad

HAPPY HERBIVORE
light & lean

OVER 150 LOW-CALORIE RECIPES
WITH WORKOUT PLANS FOR LOOKING AND FEELING GREAT

Lindsay S. Nixon

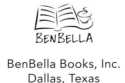

BenBella Books, Inc.
Dallas, Texas

Weight Watchers® and Points® and Points Value® are registered trademarks of Weight Watchers International, Inc. The number of Points provided here has been calculated by Lindsay Nixon based on published Weight Watchers International, Inc. information and does not imply sponsorship or endorsement of such number of Points or of this book, or recipes contained in this book, by Weight Watchers International. The *PointsPlus* value calculator on www.weightwatchers.com was used to determine the Points per serving in this cookbook. No guarantee of accuracy or warranty is given for these calculations and estimates.

Nutritional information for each recipe was computed using caloriecount.com. Each analysis provided is per serving. Unless otherwise noted, optional ingredients are not included, and when a recipe calls for multiple amounts, e.g. three to four garlic cloves, the lesser amount is computed. For nondairy milk, unsweetened almond milk was used in the calculation. Breads and buns are not included in the nutritional analysis (see packaging for that information), with the exception of wraps in the Bowls and Wraps section. Sodium content is also not included because values are significantly different between brands and because the calculator tools have too much discrepancy with sodium values to provide a safe and reliable estimate.

BenBella Books, Inc.
10300 N. Central Expressway, Suite 530
Dallas, TX 75231
www.benbellabooks.com
Send feedback to feedback@benbellabooks.com

Printed in the United States of America
10 9 8 7 6 5 4 3 2 1

Library of Congress Cataloging-in-Publication Data
Nixon, Lindsay S.
  Happy herbivore light & lean : over 150 low-calorie recipes with workout plans for looking and feeling great / by Lindsay S. Nixon.
    pages cm
  Includes bibliographical references and index.
  ISBN 978-1-937856-97-7 (pbk.) —ISBN 978-1-937856-98-4 (electronic) 1.
Reducing diets—Recipes. 2. Low-calorie diet—Recipes. 3. Vegetarian cooking. 4. Celebrity chefs. I. Title.
  RM222.2.N576 2013
  641.5'635—dc23

                              2013015471

Food photography by Jackie Sobon
Food Photography on pages 99, 107, 115, 129, 157,
    197, 230 by Neely Ross
Cover and Fitness photography and photo on page
    xvi by Matt and Natala Constantine
Recipe on page 267 by Brody's Bakery
Recipe on page 237 adapted from Goodbaker Inc.

Editing by Debbie Harmsen and Vy Tran
Copyediting by Shannon Kelly
Proofreading by Kimberly Marini and Cape Cod
    Compositors, Inc.
Cover design and interior design and
    composition by Kit Sweeney
Printed by Versa Press

Distributed by Perseus Distribution
To place orders through Perseus Distribution:
Tel: (800) 343–4499 | Fax: (800) 351–5073 | E-mail: orderentry@perseusbooks.com

Significant discounts for bulk sales are available. Please contact Glenn Yeffeth at glenn@benbellabooks.com or (214) 750–3628.

to scott & lindsey

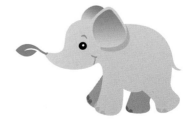

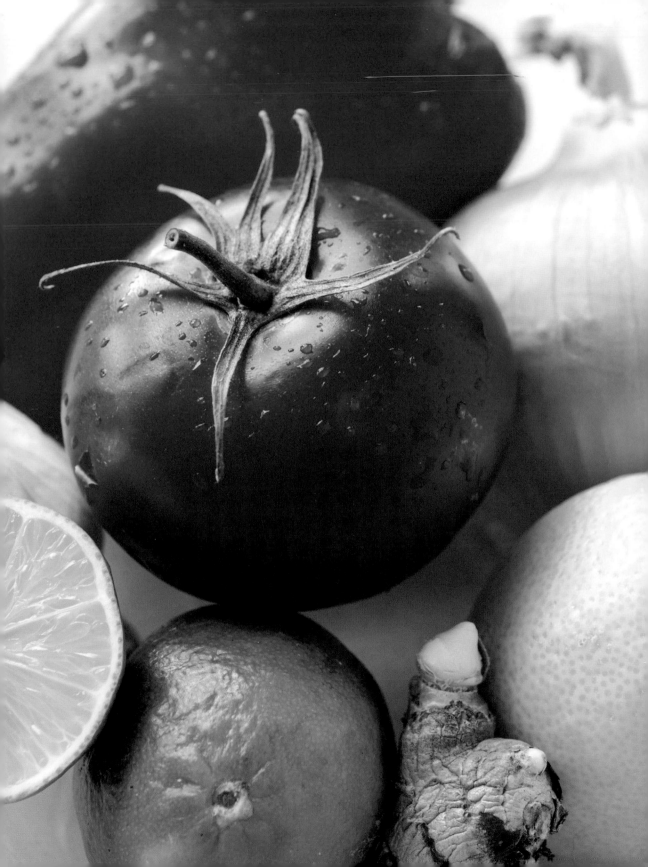

contents

by calories

Here's a rundown of every recipe in the book by its calorie count (in parentheses) and the page on which you can find it. Broths, condiments, and dressings vary in their caloric values, but the ones I have in *Happy Herbivore Light & Lean* are all fewer than 50 calories per serving.

25 CALORIES OR LESS

Balsamic-Dijon Vinaigrette (1)	137
Overnight Iced Coffee (2)	247
Vegan Worcestershire Sauce (6)	266
Ketchup (8)	261
Red Pesto (9)	156
Vegan Mayo (10)	262
Poultry Seasoning Mix (10)	268
Italian Dressing (11)	137
No-Chicken Broth Powder (12)	264
Chocolate Surprise Frosting (12)	227
Vegan Sour Cream (13)	262
Thai Peanut Dressing (19)	140
Golden Dressing (21)	141
Hummus (21)	269
Zucchini "Mozzarella" Sticks (21)	192
Chickpea "Cheese" Spread (25)	212

26–50 CALORIES

Sweet Pea Guacamole (27)	209
No-Beef Broth (27)	264
Maple Vinaigrette (30)	140
"Cheese" Ball (30)	200
Tempeh Wings (30)	204
Bloody Mary Mix (33)	251
Tofu Jerky (33)	214
Marinara Sauce (35)	263
Tempeh Bacon (36)	36
Lemony Asparagus (38)	183
Dark Chocolate Truffles (39)	230
Carol's Cabbage Soup (42)	107
AJ's Vegan Parmesan (45)	271
Brody's Gluten-Free Flour Blend (46)	267
Vegetable Broth (49)	265

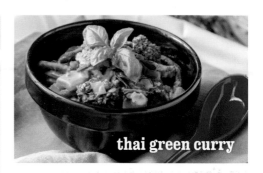

thai green curry

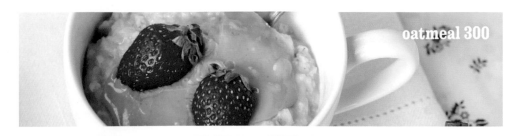

oatmeal 300

126–150 CALORIES

Quinoa Curry Cakes (128)	68
Brownies (128)	231
Chocolate Cake (128)	224
Hot Chocolate (128)	254
Chipotle Sweet Potato Salad (129)	174
Classic Cornbread (131)	55
Slow-Cooked Baked Potatoes (131)	268
Lentil Joes (131)	59
Oven Fries (131)	188
Skinny Mac 'n' Cheese (131)	150
Lentil Marinara Sauce (133)	155
Chocolate Chip Muffins (135)	44
Microwave Peach Cobbler (137)	233
Dublin (138)	248
Butternut Soup (140)	106
Skinny Cupcake (140)	240
Creamy Kale Salad (142)	180
Breakfast Tacos (145)	25
Kale Slaw (147)	177
Easy Mashed Potatoes & Gravy (147)	187
Oatmeal 300 (150)	27

151–175 CALORIES

Chipotle Pasta (152)	153
Thai Tacos (152)	64
Garden Chili (153)	120
Parmesan Greens (156)	181
Spinach Love Wrap (159)	98
Olive Gravy & Whole-Wheat Drop Biscuits (165)	33-34
Mint Mocha (166)	254
Molasses Cake (167)	221
Hungover Mary (169)	251
Smoky Apple Baked Beans (169)	172
Tempeh Burgers (169)	77

176–200 CALORIES

Mediterranean Quinoa Salad (177)	127
Yellow Curry Dal (177)	109
Chickpea Tenders (183)	63
Black & White Cookies (184)	239
Citrus Couscous (185)	184
Cream Sauce (189)	157
Pumpkin Muffin (189)	50
Jerk Tofu (193)	66
Blueberry Muffin (193)	50
Spinach & Artichoke Dip (195)	199
BBQ Wrap (200)	95
Scott's Burrito (200)	101

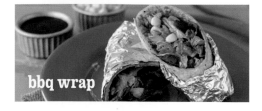

bbq wrap

201–250 CALORIES

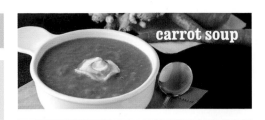

carrot soup

251–300 CALORIES

301–350 CALORIES

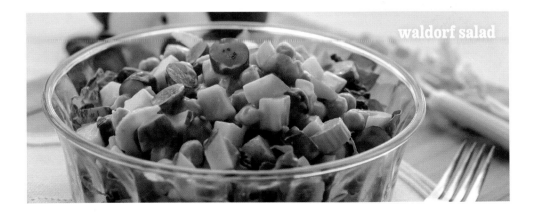

waldorf salad

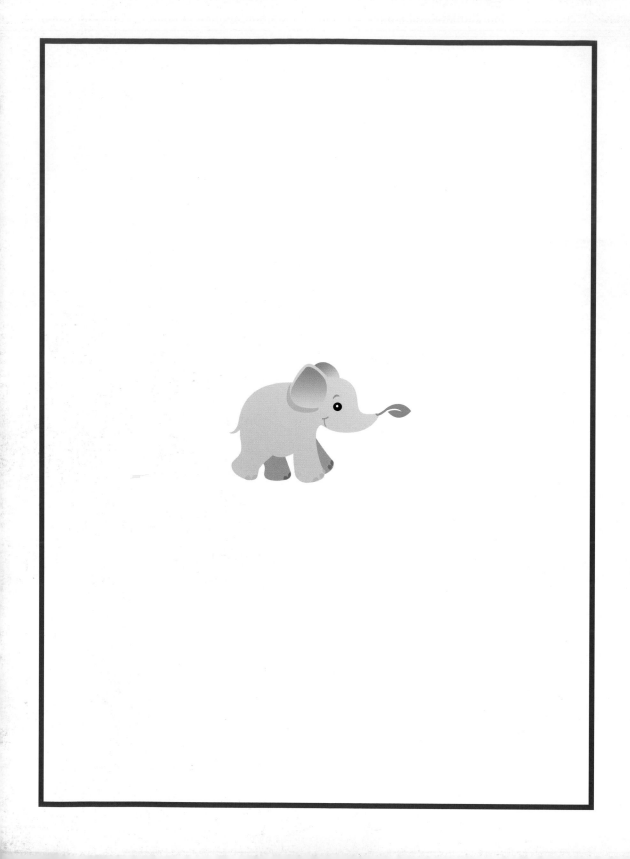

introduction

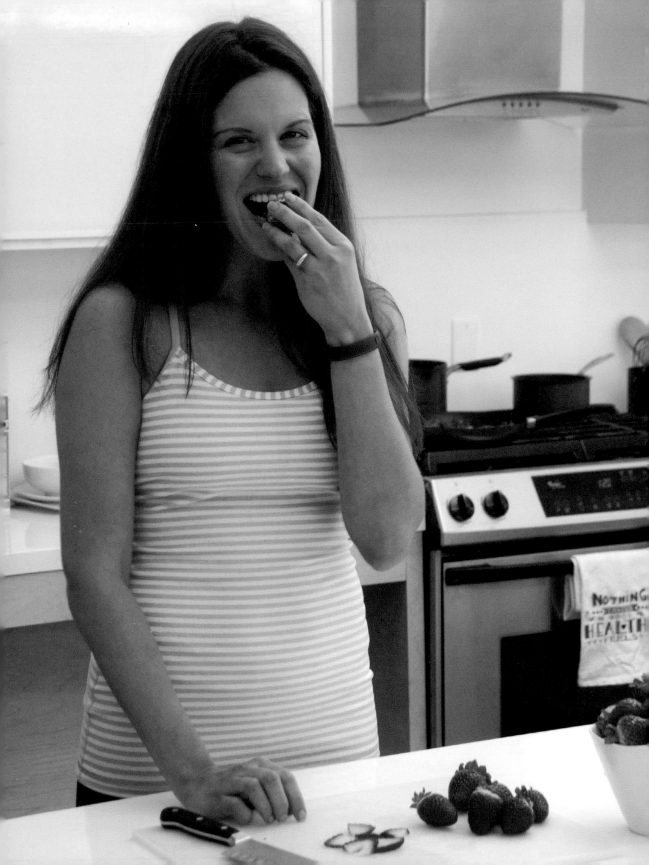

a word from lindsay

My mission with Happy Herbivore has always been to show how easy, affordable, approachable, realistic, and, most importantly, delicious, eating healthy can be.

It started with creating recipes—easy, no-fuss recipes that are built around your busy schedule (read: in 30 minutes or less) and that use normal "everyday" ingredients that you already have in your pantry or can find at your local supermarket.

But I wanted to take my mission to another level, making it even easier for you to eat healthy. I wanted to take out all of the guesswork and planning because I know from my own experiences that finding the time is often the hardest part of being healthy.

That's when I created 7-Day Meal Plans (getmealplans.com) using my no-nonsense cooking style and personal approach to eating.

Since the majority of my clients were looking to save time *and* lose weight using the meal plans, I started paying closer attention to calories—creating recipes and meals that were delicious, filling, and satisfying, while still staying within a tight calorie budget and without using any weird diet foods like artificial sweeteners. **I keep it healthy, keep it whole, keep it simple, and keep it delicious.**

Although the recipes in this cookbook are different than the recipes you'll find in the 7-Day Meal Plans, they celebrate my new "light" approach to cooking. All the recipes are 350 calories or less—but they don't scrimp on flavor or satisfaction! True to my cooking style, these recipes use only wholesome, everyday ingredients, without added fats like oil and this time, with calorie count in mind too.

And because this book is titled *Happy Herbivore Light & Lean*, I've included "recipes" for your body as well, including my basic workout and workouts that will accommodate all levels, from beginners to advanced. It's never too late to get moving!

Let's get light and lean together!

getting started

Having a supply of healthy ingredients on hand makes eating well infinitely more likely. With my 7-Day Meal Plans (getmealplans.com), I recommend that my clients make or prep their meals for the week on their day off, then reheat them throughout the week. If you multitask, making several meals at once, it only takes two to three hours to make all of your meals for the week. And if you have a healthy meal ready and waiting for you, you're less likely to be tempted to eat out or hit the drive-thru.

Even if you can't make your meals in advance, just having these ingredients on hand so you can make any meal from this book when you get home is a game changer! **Many recipes come together in less than 20 minutes.** Even a trip out of the house for "fast food" or waiting on delivery takes longer than that!

If any ingredient is unfamiliar to you, look it up in the Glossary of Ingredients (pg. 294). While most of these items should be at your local supermarket, a few items may require a trip to the health food store. You can also order many of these items online in bulk, often at a discount. My favorite bulk sites are Amazon.com, Bulkfoods.com, and Vitacost.com.

shopping list

breads & dry goods

- ☐ brown rice
- ☐ couscous
- ☐ lentils
- ☐ quinoa
- ☐ red lentils
- ☐ yellow split peas

canned goods

- ☐ black beans
- ☐ chickpeas (garbanzo beans)
- ☐ coconut milk (lite)
- ☐ green chilies
- ☐ kidney beans
- ☐ pineapple (crushed, diced)
- ☐ pumpkin (pure, *not* pumpkin pie filling)
- ☐ refried beans (vegetarian)
- ☐ tomato paste
- ☐ tomato sauce

- ☐ tomatoes (diced)
- ☐ white beans (e.g., navy beans, cannellini beans, butter beans)

condiments & dressings

- ☐ apple cider vinegar
- ☐ balsamic vinaigrette (fat-free)
- ☐ barbecue sauce
- ☐ Dijon mustard
- ☐ hot sauce (e.g., Tabasco)
- ☐ Asian hot sauce (e.g., Cholula, Sriracha)
- ☐ hummus
- ☐ ketchup
- ☐ mayonnaise (vegan; optional)
- ☐ miso (yellow or white, *not* brown)
- ☐ pineapple salsa
- ☐ salsa (regular)
- ☐ soy sauce (low sodium)*
- ☐ sweet red chili sauce
- ☐ Worcestershire sauce (vegan; optional)
- ☐ yellow mustard

soy & nondairy

- ☐ nondairy milk (e.g., soy, rice, almond)
- ☐ tempeh
- ☐ tofu (firm and extra-firm)
- ☐ vegan yogurt

fresh produce

- ☐ apples
- ☐ avocado (optional)
- ☐ baby spinach
- ☐ bananas
- ☐ basil
- ☐ bell peppers
- ☐ blueberries (or frozen)
- ☐ broccoli (or frozen)
- ☐ cabbage
- ☐ carrots
- ☐ celery
- ☐ cilantro (optional)
- ☐ cucumber
- ☐ garlic cloves
- ☐ ginger root
- ☐ grapes
- ☐ green onions
- ☐ greens (e.g., kale, collard greens, spinach)
- ☐ jalapeño
- ☐ kale
- ☐ lemons
- ☐ lettuce
- ☐ limes
- ☐ mango (or frozen)
- ☐ mint
- ☐ mushrooms
- ☐ onions
- ☐ oranges
- ☐ oregano
- ☐ potatoes
- ☐ spaghetti squash
- ☐ strawberries (or frozen)
- ☐ sweet potatoes
- ☐ thyme
- ☐ tomatoes
- ☐ zucchini

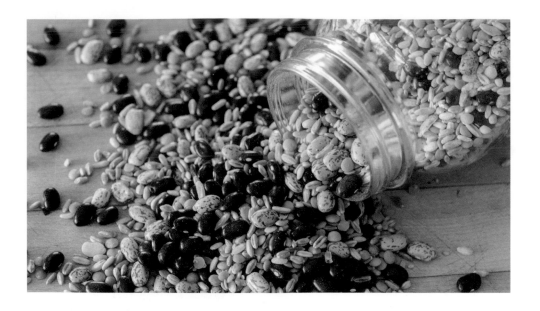

freezer

- ☐ corn
- ☐ edamame (optional)
- ☐ fruit (e.g., blueberries)
- ☐ greens (e.g., spinach)
- ☐ mixed vegetables
- ☐ nuts (optional)
- ☐ peas
- ☐ pineapple chunks
- ☐ stir-fry vegetables

pantry

- ☐ almond extract
- ☐ apple cider vinegar
- ☐ applesauce (unsweetened)
- ☐ artichoke hearts
- ☐ balsamic vinegar
- ☐ black olives
- ☐ brown rice vinegar
- ☐ dates

- ☐ green olives
- ☐ kalamata olives
- ☐ liquid smoke
- ☐ pasta (various shapes and sizes)
- ☐ noodles (whole-grain; e.g., buckwheat)
- ☐ oats (instant and rolled)
- ☐ pizza sauce or marinara sauce
- ☐ pure maple syrup
- ☐ raisins
- ☐ roasted red peppers (in water, *not* oil)
- ☐ peanut butter
- ☐ tofu (soft, shelf-stable; e.g., Mori-Nu)
- ☐ vegetable broth (low-sodium)

spices & dry herbs

- ☐ allspice
- ☐ bay leaves

- [ ] black pepper
- [ ] black salt (pg. 294)
- [ ] cayenne pepper
- [ ] chili powder
- [ ] chipotle powder
- [ ] curry powder (mild)
- [ ] dried oregano
- [ ] garam masala
- [ ] garlic powder (granulated)
- [ ] ground cinnamon
- [ ] ground coriander
- [ ] ground cumin
- [ ] ground ginger
- [ ] ground nutmeg
- [ ] Italian seasoning
- [ ] nutritional yeast
- [ ] onion flakes
- [ ] onion powder (granulated)
- [ ] paprika (regular and smoked)
- [ ] poultry seasoning (granulated, not powdered)
- [ ] pumpkin pie spice
- [ ] red pepper flakes
- [ ] rubbed sage (not powdered)
- [ ] salt
- [ ] taco seasoning (packet)
- [ ] Thai green curry paste (jar)
- [ ] Thai red curry paste (jar)
- [ ] turmeric

baking

- [ ] agave nectar (optional)
- [ ] baking powder
- [ ] baking soda
- [ ] banana extract (optional)
- [ ] brown sugar
- [ ] chocolate chips (vegan)
- [ ] chocolate extract (optional)
- [ ] confectioner's sugar
- [ ] cornmeal
- [ ] cornstarch or arrowroot
- [ ] lemon extract (optional)
- [ ] mint or peppermint extract
- [ ] molasses (not blackstrap)
- [ ] pure maple syrup
- [ ] raw sugar
- [ ] unsweetened cocoa
- [ ] vanilla extract
- [ ] vital wheat gluten*
- [ ] white whole-wheat flour

spirits & other—for drinks

- [ ] cola
- [ ] Guinness (or other stout)
- [ ] Kahlúa
- [ ] red wine
- [ ] dark rum
- [ ] sparkling water (plain and flavored)
- [ ] vodka

*gluten-free substitutes

- [ ] gluten-free all-purpose flour blend
- [ ] Orgran Gluten-Free Gluten Substitute
- [ ] gluten-free tamari

*soy-free substitutes

- [ ] chickpea miso
- [ ] coconut aminos

caloric density

A few years ago, I read two books that changed my life and approach to food forever. The first was *The Volumetrics Weight-Control Plan: Feel Full on Fewer Calories!* by Barbara Rolls and Robert A. Barnett (HarperTorch, 2000), and the second, *Mindless Eating: Why We Eat More Than We Think* by Brian Wansink (Bantam Books, 2006).

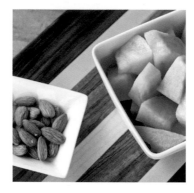

Volumetrics introduced me to the concept of caloric density or energy density—the concentration of calories in a portion of food. For example, what would leave you more satisfied: 2 tablespoons of nuts or 2 *cups* of cantaloupe? They're both approximately 106 calories. Nuts are high in caloric density while cantaloupe, like many other fruits and vegetables that are loaded with water and fiber, are much lower. Think of it another way: How fast can you eat 25 mini pretzels? Can you eat 3½ bell peppers that fast? 5 carrots? 45 celery stalks? It's hard to believe they're all roughly the same amount of calories—but they are!

If you have a voracious appetite like me, or you just like to eat a lot of food (also like me), caloric density can make a huge difference in your diet and approach to food. Caloric density is also the principle on which I base my 7-Day Meal Plans (getmealplans.com). I get more e-mails about just how *stuffed* everyone is from our big portions than I do from people who are still hungry. In fact, no one ever complains they are still hungry! Our users cannot believe how much food they can eat for 1,200+ calories.

The 7-Day Meal Plans are so filling because they center around the caloric density concept: **more food, fewer calories**. If you focus on selecting foods with a low caloric density you can worry less about how much of them you're eating *and* you'll lose weight without ever feeling hungry or deprived. It's really that simple!

Take a look at the caloric density of common foods to help put this idea in perspective (see chart on opposite page).

If you want to lose weight without scrimping on your portion size, it's clear what types of food you need to center your diet around: vegetables, fresh fruits, whole grains, and legumes. One (tricky) note: although 1 cup of garbanzo beans has about the same calories as a 5-oz serving of chicken, they don't create the same satiety. Chicken, for example, doesn't contain water or fiber, so you could easily eat two or three servings more, but you could not eat two or three servings of garbanzo beans with that same ease. These water-rich and fiber-packed foods—vegetables, whole grains, legumes, and fruits—not only help control hunger by filling you up, but they also do so on fewer calories. (Good thing those ingredients are my primary focus with the recipes in this cookbook!)

FOOD →	CALORIES
Spinach (1 cup)	7 calories
Lettuce (1 cup)	8 calories
Broccoli (1 cup)	31 calories
Carrots (1 cup)	45 calories
Strawberries (1 cup)	49 calories
Apple (1 cup)	57 calories
Pineapple (1 cup)	78 calories
Tofu (1 cup)	176 calories
Black Beans, cooked (1 cup)	210 calories
Chicken (5 oz)	214 calories
Brown Rice, cooked (1 cup)	218 calories
Lentils, cooked (1 cup)	226 calories
Beef (5 oz)	263 calories
Garbanzo Beans, cooked (1 cup)	269 calories
Oats, uncooked (1 cup)	310 calories
Raisins (1 cup)	434 calories
Flour (1 cup)	455 calories
Almonds (1 cup)	546 calories
Black Beans, uncooked (1 cup)	662 calories
Lentils, uncooked (1 cup)	678 calories
Brown rice, uncooked (1 cup)	688 calories
Garbanzo Beans, uncooked (1 cup)	728 calories
Sugar (1 cup)	774 calories
Cashews (1 cup)	786 calories
Olive Oil (1 cup)	1,728 calories

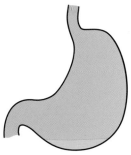

400 calories of oil

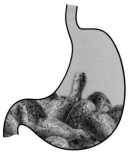

400 calories of chicken

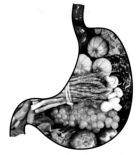

400 calories of vegetables

the 100 factor—calories

I did not wake up one morning 40 pounds heavier. The weight crept up gradually, seemingly unnoticed over several years. Although my diet wasn't perfect, I wasn't binging on cheesecake or ice cream, or eating greasy fast food very often. In other words, I wasn't engaging in any of the behaviors that I assumed I needed to do in order to gain weight.

After reading *Mindless Eating: Why We Eat More Than We Think* by Brian Wansink, I finally understood how I'd gained weight and why many of us do without noticing. You don't need to be binging on junk food. You don't even need to be binging.

100 CALORIES. THAT'S ALL IT TAKES.

You can lose 10 pounds a year by simply shaving off 100 calories per day—that's one tablespoon of mayonnaise, a slice of bread, one tablespoon of peanut butter, or six crackers. It doesn't take much. On the flip side, you need to only exceed your daily calorie needs by 100 calories to *gain* 10 pounds a year.

Here's how it works:

By leaving out 100 calories per day, you are eating 36,500 fewer calories a year (100 calories/day x 365 days = 36,500 calories). It takes a deficit of 3,500 calories to lose 1 pound of fat, so a deficit of 36,500 works out to a little more than 10 pounds of lost fat.

On the flip side, by overeating 100 calories per day, you are eating an additional 36,500 calories a year. Divide 36,500 by 3,500 (the amount of calories in 1 pound of fat) and you end up with 10.4 pounds—a (more than) 10-pound weight gain per year. Go one step further and multiply that by 10 years and that's more than 100 extra pounds!

According to Wansink, on a day-to-day basis we "wouldn't know if we ate 200 or 300 calories more or less than the day before. . . . If we eat too little, we know

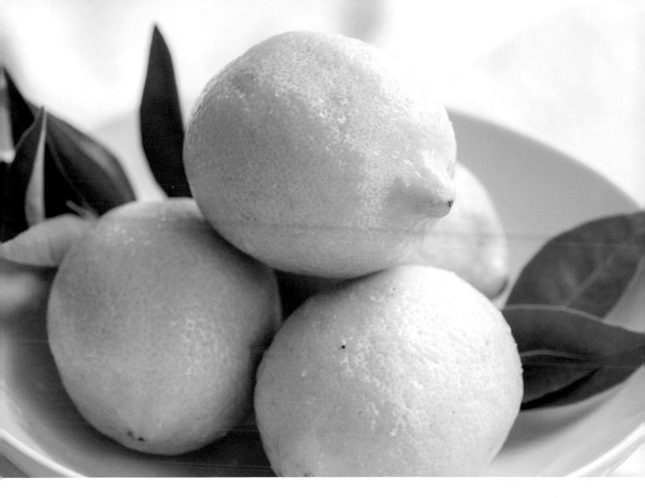

it. If we eat way too much, we know it. But there is a calorie range—a mindless margin—where we feel fine and are unaware of small differences. That is, the difference between 1,900 calories and 2,000 calories is one we cannot detect, nor can we detect the difference between 2,000 and 2,100 calories. But over the course of a year, this mindless margin would either cause us to lose ten pounds or gain ten pounds."

Shaving 100 calories off is easy, especially if you start choosing foods based on caloric density. You can also shed an extra 10 pounds a year by burning an extra 100 calories a day with movement—riding a bike for 10 minutes, walking for 30 minutes on your lunch break, cleaning your house, etc. (See the Lean section for 42 ways to burn 100 calories, pg. 279)

If you do both—shave 100 calories off your food and slip in a tiny bit of exercise—you'll lose 20 pounds a year pretty effortlessly. *Now that's light and lean!*

my journey to health

Fans and the media frequently ask me about my "story": my personal journey to health. Over the years I've given away bits and pieces, but I've never really sat down and spelled it all out—told the whole story. I guess a part of me was always shy about it. *Am I ready to share my deepest, darkest thoughts and personal insecurities out loud?* I decided with this book, now is the time.

I can remember the day I became self-conscious with my body. I was a child, about eight years old or so, at a pool party in the two-piece bathing suit I'd persuaded my mom to buy me. (She insisted I was much too young for one, but I insisted all the girls my age were wearing them and putting water balloons in their tops to look like they had boobs.)

I was so excited to be wearing that two-piece. It hardly showed my stomach at all, but I felt cool, like a *teenager*. I was sitting on the patio, noshing on watermelon, feeling awesome as ever when an adult at the party pointed out all my fat rolls.

Looking back at old photos, I don't think I was ever a chubby kid, but I wasn't particularly slender either. I probably would have been slimmer if I had been physically active. As a child I had more of an active mind than an active body. While other kids played sports, I wrote poems and short stories. Maybe you could say I had a little "pudge" or baby fat. The point is, from that day forward I became self-conscious about how I looked. I'm in my 30s now, and I still look down when I sit in a bikini.

But I'm a success story. I lost that baby fat (and the adult fat I gained too). After years of struggling and torturing myself with myriad diets and the latest exercise fads, I finally found a solution—a real solution. I lost the weight and kept it off (easily!) when I adopted a low-fat, plant-based diet. I also changed my relationship with food, as well as my relationship with eating and "dieting," and that's the success I'm most proud of. That's the success I hope to give you by sharing my story—my journey—to real health.

I grew up a vegetarian largely out of a love for animals. When I was seven, I was eating a hamburger as we drove past grazing cows, put two and two together,

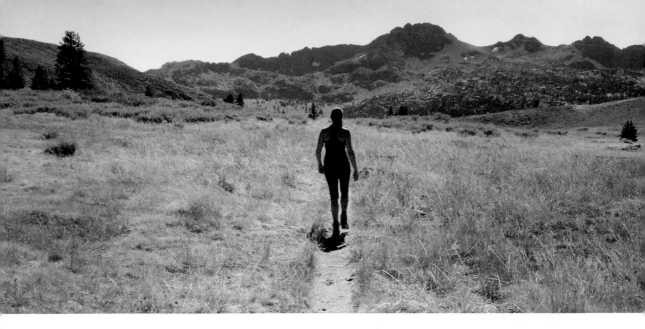

and that was that. I fell out of my vegetarian ways in my teen years from peer pressure and familial pressure, and my health started to decline immediately. I developed acne and constant, crippling migraines. I also gained weight. My doctor chalked it all up to puberty.

Being a teenager in Florida was exciting but hard because I had to be in a bathing suit year-round among my peers. I masked my insecurities by acting confident and a bit egotistical. Secretly I hated my thighs and love handles and cursed my beautiful girlfriends who had such skinny, "perfect" bodies. *Why them and not me?*

In college, I lived a busy life: work, class, extracurricular activities, boy-friends—and between my hectic schedule and being broke, I missed meals pretty often (unintentionally). I slimmed down noticeably in the first year and loved all the attention and compliments my new body was getting me. For the first time in my life, my friends were jealous of *me.*

This continued until my senior year when I met my now husband. A few weeks after we started dating, Scott made a passing comment that when we first went out, he thought I was anorexic and didn't eat. I was mortified. I hadn't ordered much food on our first date (or second, or third!) because I was so ner-vous and I felt bad that he—someone who also was struggling financially—was graciously paying for my meals. But then I became worried he wouldn't like me because I'd been peckish, and I already liked him so much. So I made a point to eat. I sort of let loose and ate foods with abandon. I wasn't binging or gorging, I was just eating (and drinking) whatever I wanted without pausing to figure out what the healthiest option was. If I gained weight, I told myself it wouldn't matter, Scott would love me anyway.

By the time our first anniversary rolled around, both of us were the chubbiest we'd ever been in our entire lives. What's the saying? We were fat and happy.

Scott and I met in January and the following fall, I can distinctly remember pulling my winter clothes from the closest and being baffled—truly baffled—why none of them fit. I kept trying them on and wondering what the problem was. *How did all my clothes shrink in the closet?* I just wore them eight months ago! Never did the thought occur to me that I had put on substantial weight. No, no. I was the same. I continued to live in my denial until a serious health scare changed everything.

Just as I had been in college, in law school I was busy, juggling a full-time job, classes, my studies, and my long-distance boyfriend. I knew I needed to go to the doctor for a regular exam, but I just couldn't find the time. Besides, I was in my early 20s and healthy. *What was the big rush? I wasn't dying!*

Eventually I found the time to go (truthfully, I'd run out of migraine pills and knew I couldn't get more without a new prescription). When the exam was over, I knew something was wrong. If everything is perfect, doctors don't ask you with a worried look to come back as soon as possible.

It turned out that my cervix had visitors: precancerous cells—and a lot of them. I was shocked. How could I face cancer at such a young age when my whole life was still ahead of me? Thankfully, the doctor detected it early enough that the cells could be removed without much disturbance to my life, and so they were. But the entire experience (and procedure!) rattled me. It was my wake-up call.

Just a few years earlier, my grandmother had died—no, she wasted away painfully and slowly—of cancer, and I refused to have the same fate. Cancer wasn't going to happen to me again, I resolved. I got busy making changes: I joined a gym. I started cooking meals rather than eating out. I started reading books on nutrition. Before long, I found myself migrating back to the vegetarian diet of my childhood. I thought being a vegetarian would help me make better food choices, and it did. I started to lose weight and generally feel better.

About a year later I went vegan as an experiment. I'd heard that a vegan diet was great for weight loss and I still had weight to lose. I'd also heard that going vegan could clear up your skin, and after a decade of embarrassing acne, I was willing to try anything. There were other motivations, too. I'd become increasingly more aware of the plight of farm animals and the ecological consequences of animal products, so on a trip to San Francisco—a town known for being vegan-friendly—I gave it a whirl.

I decided to stick with my new diet after returning home to Boston, but I was also worried about my health—*where would I get my protein and calcium*, I wondered. I started reading more books. I read *Skinny Bitch*[1] and *The China Study*[2], two books that solidified my decision to adopt a 100 percent plant-based diet and take it one step further: I eliminated oil and most added fats, and I focused on eating whole foods.

My world changed. I lost weight quickly and effortlessly. I started sleeping better. My acne went away and so did the stomach issues that I thought were "normal." My migraines were all but nonexistent. I had so much energy that 10 months after adopting my new diet, I ran a marathon even though I was too out of shape to walk a 5K the year before. I started snowboarding and mountain biking—two sports that had previously seemed so extreme and beyond my reach.

Those around me took notice. Friends asked my secret. Strangers asked how I got my glow or my long, shiny hair. It was like that time in college all over, except this time I'd achieved my healthy appearance in a wholesome way.

Still, there was a part of me—that self-conscious part—that was terrified I'd gain all the weight back. So I went to the gym. A lot. For a few years, I was a bit of a gym rat. I had to go five days a week to feel sane. Sometimes I went seven days a week. I liked working out and being at the gym so much that I became a personal trainer.

Then something happened. I don't know how or why exactly, but I lost my gym mojo. It was gradual, but before long I was going so infrequently that I started to think I should cancel my gym membership—but that *scared* me. If I

---

1 *Skinny Bitch: A No-Nonsense, Tough-Love Guide for Savvy Girls Who Want To Stop Eating Crap and Start Looking Fabulous!* Rory Freedman and Kim Barnouin. Running Press, 2005.
2 *The China Study: The Most Comprehensive Study of Nutrition Ever Conducted and the Startling Implications for Diet, Weight Loss, and Long-Term Health.* Colin T. Campbell, PhD, and Thomas M. Campbell II, BenBella Books, 2006.

canceled, then I wouldn't go at all, and what would happen to my midsection? So I kept the membership, hoping it would motivate me to go back to the gym.

Eventually life got in the way. We moved abroad to the Caribbean and a gym membership wasn't an option. Our new apartment complex had a gym, but it was tiny—two treadmills, an elliptical, and some free weights. I'd go sometimes, but not regularly. There were a few months in which I didn't go at all.

A year later we moved back to the States, to Colorado. I told myself I didn't need to go to the gym because I'd be snowboarding all the time. And I did snow-board pretty often, a few days a week. Usually for a few hours of time (but a lot of that time involved sitting on my butt on the lift), and given our unseasonably dry and warm winter that year, some weeks we didn't get any snow and I didn't go at all. So in reality, I wasn't much more active than I had been on the island.

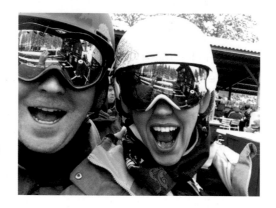

At this point I had spent two years without really exercising or stepping foot into a gym. Realizing this, I decided to get back into working out and joined a gym when we moved to California. Part of the gym orientation involved meeting with a trainer for a fitness evaluation. I dreaded it for days, but when I finally mustered the courage to go I was delighted to see that after two years, my weight/BMI was still in the low end of the healthy range for my height, and my body fat percentage was also in the low end of average. And, worried about those old midsection rolls (where everything started!), I looked down to check: I had no more rolls than when I was working out almost daily.

Finally, I had found my balance. I'd found what worked for me. Even in a period of inactivity, I'd become able to keep my weight—and my health—in check. It wasn't a vanity diet. It wasn't a diet that required me to exercise excessively. I just had to keep myself naturally active and eat right. Eat a low-fat, whole-foods diet. It's that diet—and that balance—that I'm celebrating in this cookbook.

how to use the icons

- ✔ **QUICK** Recipes that come together in 30 minutes or less. Some recipes may require multitasking to complete in 30 minutes.

- ✔ **FAT-FREE** Recipes with less than 1 gram of fat per serving.

- ✔ **GLUTEN-FREE** Recipes that don't require whole-wheat flour, vital wheat gluten, or barley. I can't vouch for all the ingredients, so if you have an allergy or sensitivity, please make sure every ingredient you use is certified gluten-free. Gluten-free tamari or Coconut Aminos may be used in place of soy sauce, and Orgran makes a gluten-free gluten substitute that can replace vital wheat gluten. In baking recipes calling for whole-wheat flour, you may use a gluten-free all-purpose blend (see pg. 267 for a recipe). Note that while oats themselves do not contain gluten, they may be cross-contaminated. Use a certified gluten-free variety of oats for your safety.

- ✔ **SOY-FREE** Recipes that don't require tofu, soy sauce, tempeh, or other soy products. If the recipe calls for nondairy milk, use almond milk or rice milk. If a recipe calls for vegan yogurt, use almond, coconut, or rice-based vegan yogurt instead of soy yogurt. Also, use chickpea miso for recipes calling for miso, and Coconut Aminos can replace soy sauce or tamari.

- ✔ **BUDGET** Recipes that cost $5 or less to prepare with a well-stocked pantry and spice rack.

- ✔ **PANTRY** Recipes that can be made using only pantry ingredients, spices, and condiments, plus a few fresh pantry staples like onions, garlic, ginger, potatoes, and citrus fruits. Canned equivalents are suitable for the frozen or fresh ingredients in the Pantry recipes. Some recipes using fresh basil are classified as Pantry recipes, since many of us keep basil plants in our kitchen or garden.

- ✔ **SINGLE SERVING** Recipes that serve one or make only one item, for example, one wrap.

LIGHT

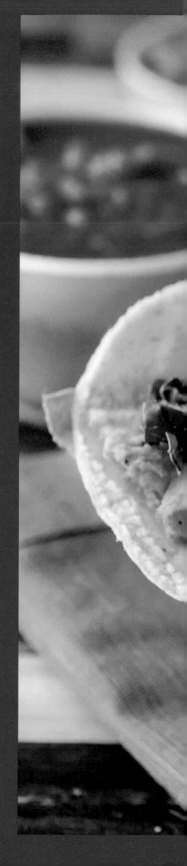

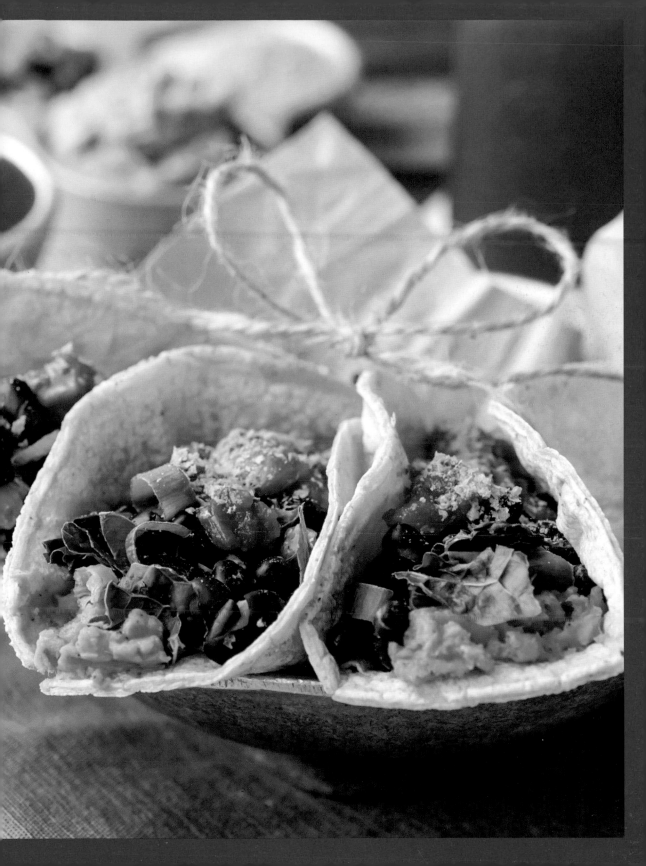

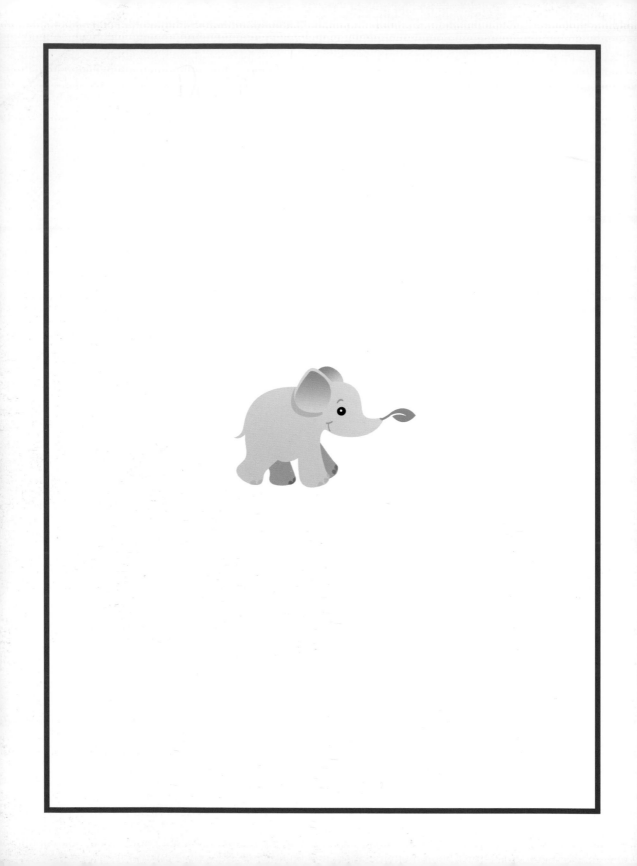

breakfast

pumpkin pancakes

PER PANCAKE
(WITHOUT TOPPINGS)

Calories 89
Fat. 0.8g
Carbs 18.3g
Sugars. 1g
Fiber 1.1g
Protein 2.4g
WW Points. 2

MAKES 6

- 1 c white whole-wheat flour
- 1 tbsp baking powder
- ½ tsp pumpkin pie spice
- pinch salt
- 4 tbsp pure pumpkin (canned)
- 1 c nondairy milk (any flavor)
- 1 tbsp brown sugar (optional)
- pure maple syrup (for dipping)

Come fall, I love anything that has pumpkin in it. I'm a sucker for the pumpkin flavoring, but I also feel good about slipping squash into my food. This means that any recipe of mine that can get a little pumpkin love does—including my pancakes!

In a mixing bowl, whisk flour with baking powder, pumpkin pie spice, and salt until well combined. Stir in pure pumpkin, nondairy milk, and sugar if using. Let batter rest for 10 minutes. Meanwhile, heat a nonstick skillet. When a drop of water fizzles on the skillet, it's ready. Turn heat down to low and pour pancake batter into skillet, ¼ cup at a time. Cook on one side until bubbles form, about 2 minutes, then gently flip it over and cook another 2–3 minutes. Repeat until you are out of batter. Dip in maple syrup, if desired.

They say breakfast is the most important meal of the day. Personally, I like breakfast foods best at dinner, and pancakes, especially, are good at any time of the day.

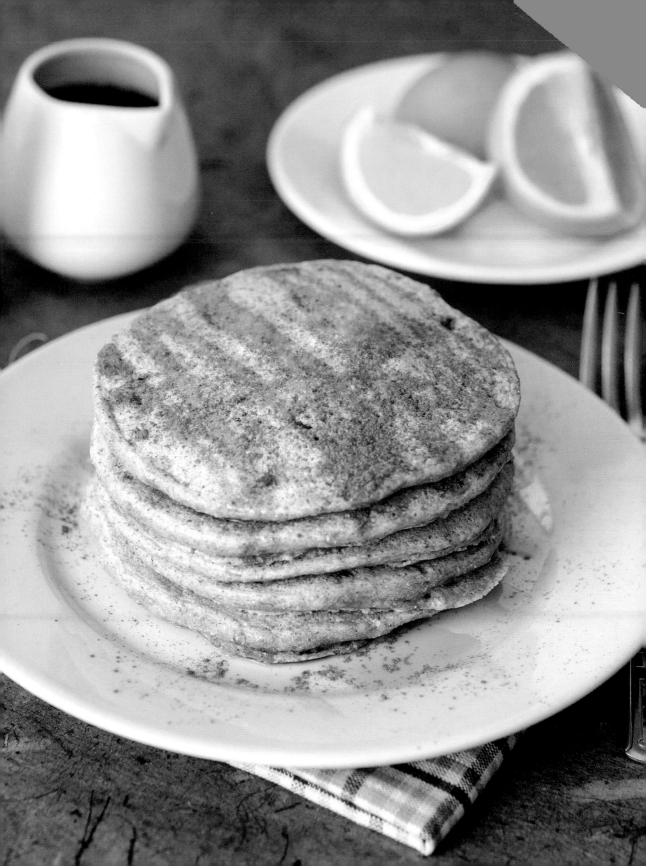

Delish!

PER PANCAKE
(WITHOUT TOPPINGS)

Calories 94
Fat. 0.7g
Carbs 19.8g
Fiber 1g
Sugars. 1.9g
Protein 2.4g
WW Points 2

MAKES 6

- 1 c white whole-wheat flour
- 1 tbsp baking powder
- pinch salt
- ground ginger (optional)
- 1 c nondairy milk (plain or vanilla)
- 2 tbsp pineapple juice (from the can) or water
- 1–2 tbsp raw sugar (optional)
- ½ c chopped pineapple
- toppings

made c mom, dad when in MH 1st trip to new house 4/14

pineapple pancakes

If pancakes and pineapple upside-down cake had a baby... I like to eat these pancakes topped with more pineapple juice (it makes the pancakes soggy like a sponge cake), applesauce, or vanilla vegan yogurt. Pure maple syrup would also work.

In a mixing bowl, whisk flour, baking powder, salt, and a few dashes of ground ginger (if using) together. Add nondairy milk and pineapple juice (or water), and stir to combine. For a sweeter pancake, you can add 1–2 tbsp raw sugar. Let batter rest 10 minutes. If it's too thick, add more nondairy milk or water. Heat non-stick skillet. When it's hot (a drop of water will sizzle), reduce heat to low and pour in ¼ cup of batter. Add a few chopped pineapple pieces on top of each pancake, cook until bubbles form, about 2 minutes, then gently flip it over and cook another minute or two.

Chef's Notes

» I find that ground ginger really makes pineapple sparkle. You can also add a drop of coconut extract for a little Hawaiian flair.

» Diced pineapple (canned or frozen) is usually too big. You might need to chop it up more for this recipe.

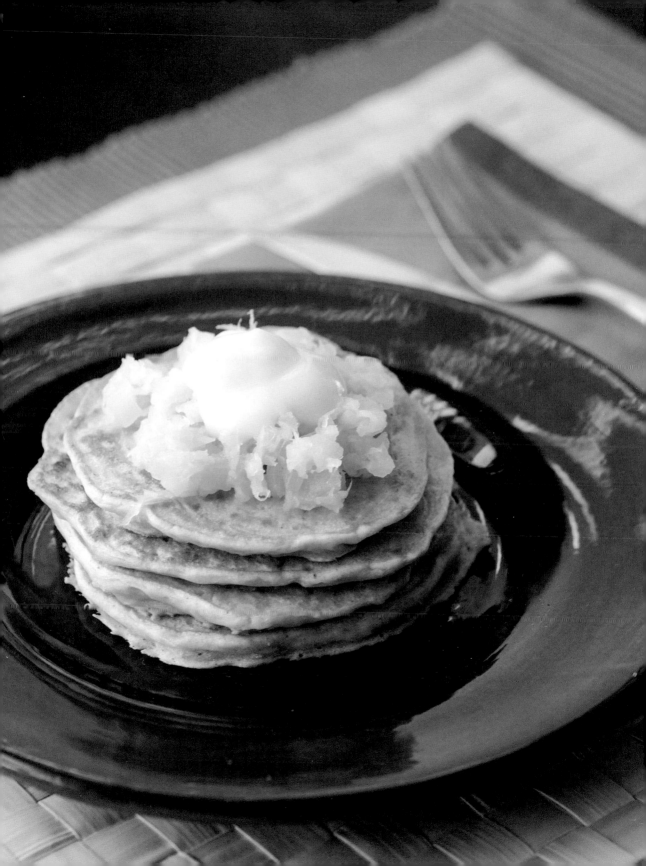

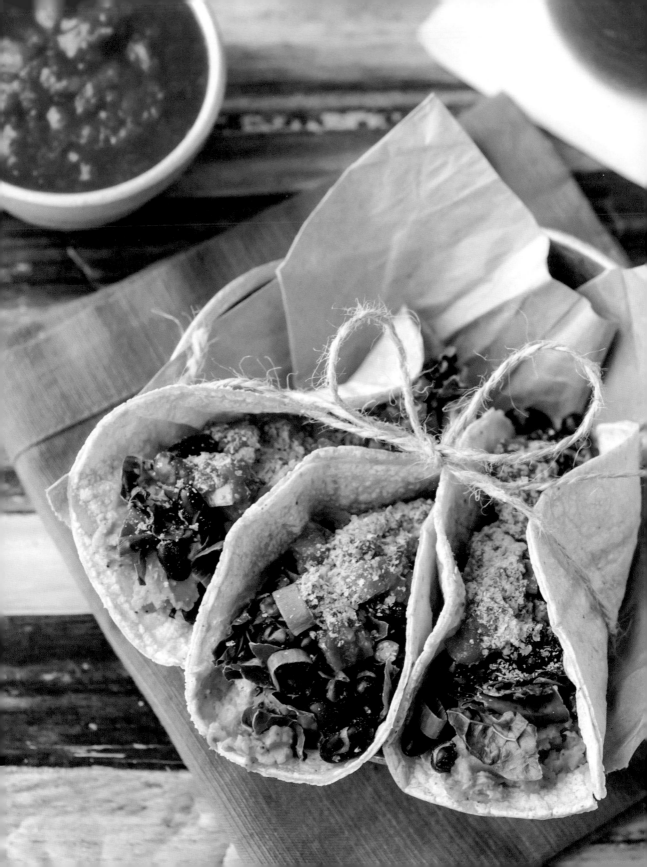

breakfast tacos

I'm always looking for ways to slip more vegetables into my diet (particularly at breakfast) and these tacos hit the nail on the head: greens, beans, and sweet potatoes before lunch? I can feel good about that! Bonus: They are really filling and leave me satisfied for hours. I tend to make these tacos for breakfast when I have leftover cooked greens and sweet potatoes from the day before.

Warm corn tortillas if they've been in your fridge. I like to heat each side over a low flame for 10–15 seconds on my gas stove, but a few seconds in the microwave covered with a damp paper towel also works. Mash sweet potato with a fork (you can mix in spices like ground cumin, chili powder, garlic powder, onion powder, and cayenne if you like, or even a basic fajita or taco seasoning with a splash of nondairy milk) and spread into the center of the tortilla. Top with beans, greens, and green onions, plus hot sauce, salsa, nutritional yeast, and guacamole as desired (I overflow my tacos so they are really filled). Enjoy!

PER TACO

Calories	145
Fat	1.3g
Carbs	29.1g
Fiber	5.6g
Sugars	3g
Protein	5.2g
WW Points	4

MAKES 3

- 3 corn tortillas
- 1 sweet potato, cooked
- ½ c cooked black beans
- ½ c cooked greens (e.g., steamed kale or collards)
- 2 green onions, sliced
  hot sauce
  salsa (optional)
  nutritional yeast (optional)
  guacamole (optional)

Chef's Note Make a "taco bar" and serve these for brunch when you have a big crowd. Tofu Scramble (pg. 35) is another great filling option.

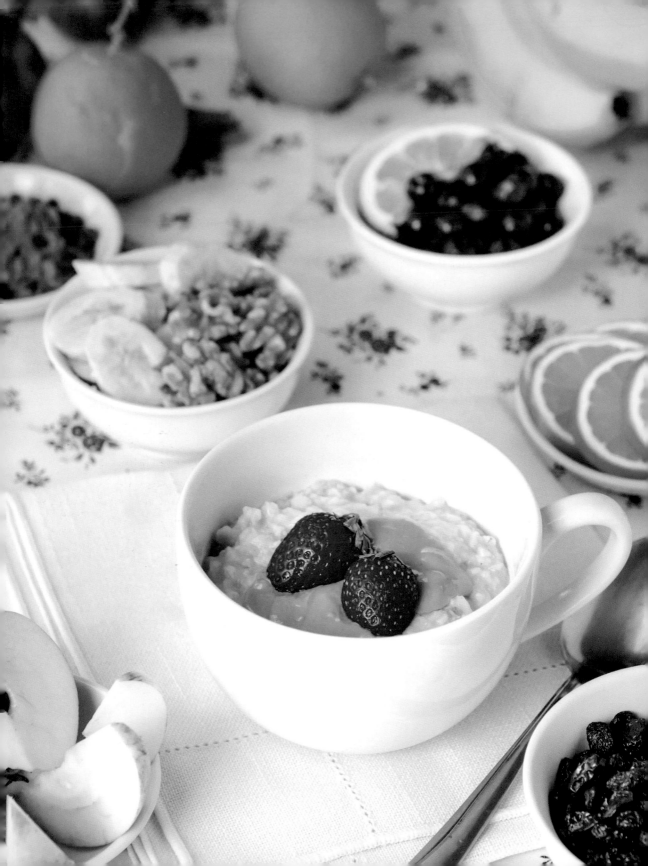

oatmeal 300

It's no secret that oatmeal is a healthy breakfast. I wanted to like oatmeal, I really did, but it was just so *meh*. I'd find myself dumping peanut butter or sugar on top just to get it down and then my oatmeal was more like a candy bar than a healthy breakfast. I'd given up on liking oatmeal until I started selling my 7-Day Meal Plans (getmealplans.com). Knowing how many people loved oatmeal, I set out to create oatmeal recipes that were so flavorful and exciting that even *I* would want to eat them. Here is the basic recipe for oatmeal followed by some of my favorite combinations—all for 300 calories or less!

Combine oats and water in a small saucepan, adding more water if you like your oatmeal to be a little soupy. (If using frozen, dried, or fresh fruits, add with oats and water.) Bring to a boil, reduce heat to medium, and continue to cook, stirring regularly, until you have oatmeal. Add remaining ingredients (see add-ons), stir to combine, and then garnish.

PER BOWL
(WITHOUT ADD-ONS)

Calories 150
Fat. 3g
Carbs 27g
Fiber 4g
Sugars 1g
Protein 5g
WW Points 4

SINGLE SERVING

½ c rolled oats
¾ c water

Chef's Notes

» You can add a little nondairy milk at the end for creamier oatmeal.

» While oats themselves are gluten-free, many brands are cross-contaminated. If you have an allergy or sensitivity, please purchase certified gluten-free oats.

SEE NEXT PAGE FOR RECIPE ADD-ONS »

OATMEAL ADD-ONS

APPLE PIE

½ apple, diced
ground cinnamon (to taste)
¼ c unsweetened applesauce
2 tbsp brown sugar, or 1¼ tbsp maple
    syrup (garnish)
Calories: 298

BANANA BREAD

¼ c unsweetened applesauce
drop or two vanilla extract
ground cinnamon
dash ground nutmeg
½ banana, sliced (garnish)
1¼ tbsp walnuts or pecans (garnish)
Calories: 296

BLUEBERRY MUFFIN

¼ c unsweetened applesauce
1⅓ c frozen blueberries
1 tsp lemon zest, or to taste
Calories: 293

CHERRY-VANILLA

1 c pitted cherries (frozen)
vanilla extract (to taste)
1 tbsp brown sugar or 1¾ tsp maple
    syrup (garnish)
3 tbsp unsweetened applesauce
Calories: 300

CHOCOLATE-CHOCOLATE

2 tbsp unsweetened cocoa
1 tbsp unsweetened applesauce
ground cinnamon (optional)
½ banana, sliced (garnish)
1 tbsp chocolate chips (garnish)
Calories: 296

CINNAMON RAISIN

3 tbsp raisins (soak in hot water
    10 minutes)
¼ c unsweetened applesauce
2 tsp pure maple syrup (garnish)
ground cinnamon (to taste)
Calories: 297

ORANGE SCENTED

¾ c orange juice (instead of water)
1 tsp orange zest (or to taste)
⅔ orange, sliced, or blueberries
    (garnish)
Calories: 284

PEANUT BUTTER

¼ c unsweetened applesauce
3¼ tsp peanut butter (garnish)
2 strawberries, sliced (garnish)
Calories: 298

PUMPKIN PIE

¼ c pure pumpkin (canned)
¼ tsp pumpkin pie spice
2 tbsp raisins
1¼ tbsp pure maple syrup (garnish)
Calories: 297

RASPBERRY CREME

½ c frozen raspberries
½ banana, sliced
2 oz vegan yogurt, preferably vanilla
    (garnish)
Calories: 290

oatmeal pancakes

If you've made too much oatmeal (pg. 27), here is the answer for your leftovers. What I love most about these pancakes is how hearty they are. I'm filled up after two or three, and they stick with me for hours.

In a blender or mini food processor, blend banana with water and set aside. In a mixing bowl, whisk flour and baking powder together, plus a few dashes of pumpkin pie spice or ground cinnamon. Add banana-water mixture and stir a few times. Add oatmeal and stir again, adding ¼ cup nondairy milk. If it's really thick, add another 1–2 tbsp liquid. Heat a nonstick skillet over high heat. When a water droplet sizzles, it's ready. Reduce heat slightly (to medium-high) and pour in ¼ cup of batter, using the back of the measuring cup to flatten and expand the pancake a little (so there is not a big mound in the center). When the pancake is filled with bubbles (after about a minute), slide a nonstick spatula under and flip it over. Let it cook another 2 minutes, pressing down on the pancake with the spatula a few times. Flip over again for about 15–30 seconds. Top with applesauce, maple syrup, or fresh fruit.

PER PANCAKE

Calories 97
Fat 0.8g
Carbs 19.9g
Fiber 1.7g
Sugars 1.5g
Protein 2.8g
WW Points 2

MAKES 9

- 1 small ripe banana
- ¾ c water
- 1 c white whole-wheat flour
- 2 tsp baking powder
- pumpkin pie spice or ground cinnamon
- 1 c leftover oatmeal
- ¼ c nondairy milk (plain or vanilla)
- toppings

Chef's Note Do not stack these pancakes. They will steam and become soggy.

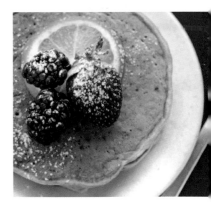

PER SERVING
(ABOUT ¼ CUP)

Calories 107
Fat. 2.1g
Carbs 19.7g
Fiber 2.3g
Sugars. 5.9g
Protein 2.9g
WW Points 3

MAKES 2½ CUPS

2⅓ c rolled oats

1 tsp ground cinnamon

⅓ c unsweetened applesauce

¼ c pure maple syrup

1–2 tbsp smooth peanut butter

1 tsp banana extract or vanilla extract

⅓ c raisins (optional)

Chef's Note If, after 30 minutes of baking, your granola is still soft and not crisp, spread it out thinly on a cookie sheet lined with parchment paper and bake a few minutes more. If the granola is packed together or overlapping, it won't crisp.

granola

I'm always getting e-mail requests for a low-fat granola recipe and after browsing the nutritional information of granola at the grocery store, I saw why! At only 107 calories a serving, this low-fat (oil-free!) granola is one you can feel good about. I love to put it on top of vegan yogurt, but it's a great snack, too!

Preheat oven to 300°F. Line a jelly roll pan or cookie sheet with parchment paper or use a large, rectangular (9x13) glass casserole dish and set aside. In a mixing bowl, combine oats and ground cinnamon. In a small bowl or measuring cup, whisk applesauce, maple syrup, peanut butter, and extract together until well combined. Pour over oats and use a spatula to combine the mixture, evenly coating all the oats. Transfer mixture to your prepared pan or dish, spreading it out, and bake 10 minutes. Stir well, breaking up any large chunks with the spatula, and bake another 10 minutes. Stir again and bake another 5–10 minutes, or until golden and crisp, like granola. (Note: The granola firms and crisps slightly as it cools.) Mix in raisins, if using, after baking. Store granola in an airtight container, preferably at room temperature.

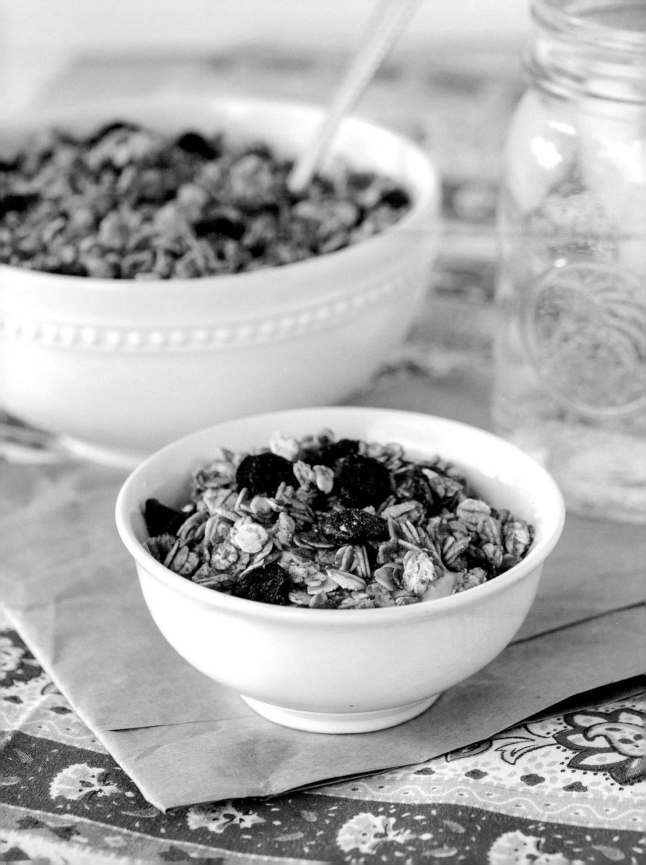

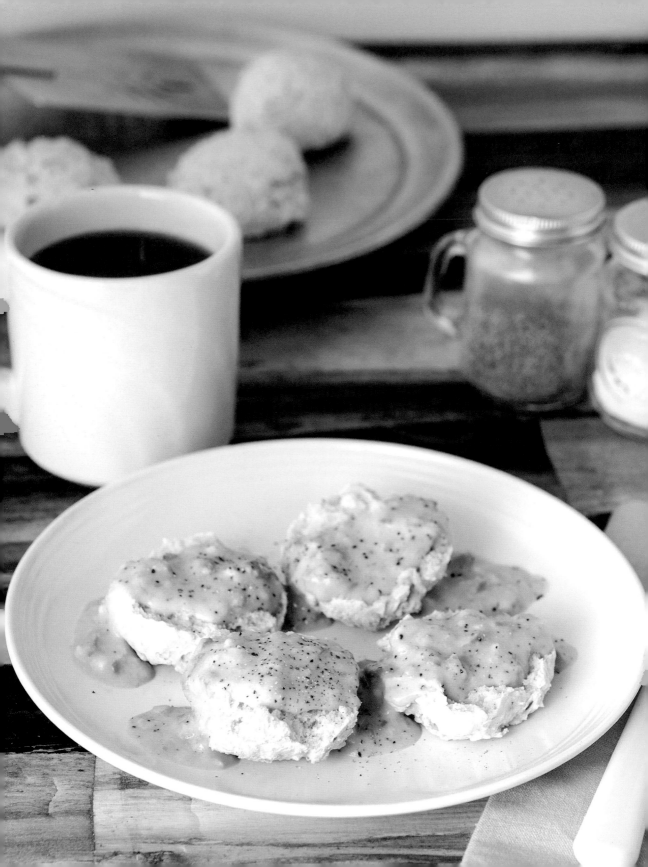

whole-wheat drop biscuits

Here are my quick-n-easy whole-wheat drop biscuits. For brunch, try smothering these biscuits with the Olive Gravy (pg. 34) with a side of Tempeh Bacon (pg. 36) and/or Tofu Scramble (pg. 35), spinach, and olives. These biscuits are also a nice complement to dinner and really stick with you.

Preheat oven to 425°F. Line a cookie sheet with parchment paper and set aside. In a large mixing bowl, whisk flour, baking powder, and salt together. Stir in applesauce, so it makes large clumps. A light flour dusting is okay, but make sure there are no hidden flour pockets at the bottom. Pour in nondairy milk, gently stirring until a wet, thick, doughy batter forms. Add an extra splash of liquid if necessary. Drop five spoonfuls on your cookie sheet, leaving space between them. For round biscuits, use clean fingers to smooth out each drop into a circular shape. Bake 7–10 minutes or until the biscuits are firm to the touch and golden around the edges.

PER BISCUIT

Calories 93
Fat 0.4g
Carbs 19.4g
Fiber 2.6g
Sugars 2.5g
Protein 3.6g
WW Points 2

MAKES 5

1 c white whole-wheat flour
1 tsp baking powder
pinch salt
¼ c unsweetened applesauce
¼ c nondairy milk

olive gravy

PER SERVING
[ABOUT ¼ CUP]

Calories 72
Fat. 2.4g
Carbs 10g
Fiber 3g
Sugars. 0.5g
Protein 4.4g
WW Points 2

SERVES 3

vegetable broth

3 garlic cloves, minced

¼ c chopped green olives

½ tsp onion powder

½ c nondairy milk

2 tbsp white whole-wheat or brown rice flour

2 tbsp nutritional yeast

black pepper, to taste

juice from 2 lemon slices

Whole-Wheat Drop Biscuits (pg. 33)

Chef's Note For a gluten-free version, use brown rice flour.

I usually serve this savory gravy over Whole-Wheat Drop Biscuits (pg. 33), but it's a great alternative that you can use any way you'd normally use gravy—on mashed potatoes, beans, grains, vegetables, etc.

Line a saucepan with a thin layer of broth and sauté garlic and green olives until garlic is golden and broth has evaporated. Add onion powder and stir. In a measuring cup, whisk nondairy milk with flour and nutritional yeast. Pour over olive mixture and heat over high. Once it's nearly boiling, reduce heat to low and continue to stir as it thickens. Add a generous amount of black pepper to taste, plus lemon juice. If it gets too thick, add more nondairy milk.

Pictured on page 32 with the Whole-Wheat Drop Biscuits.

tofu scramble

I think some variation of this tofu scramble ends up in every one of my cookbooks and for good reason: It's cheap, fast, easy, highly adaptable, satisfying, and fairly low in calories. Adding in your leftover greens, vegetables, beans, etc., extends the dish and makes it more satisfying. My best friend Jim, for example, is always adding frozen mixed vegetables to his scramble, which extends the servings from two to four, and gives you the good feeling of eating veggies at breakfast! You can also make a big batch once and reheat it for days. (I've also been known to eat it cold, particularly in a wrap, "burrito" style.)

Drain tofu and mash in a skillet with a potato masher (or crumble with your hands). Stir in all ingredients from nutritional yeast to turmeric and cook over high heat, adding a splash of water or nondairy milk to prevent sticking if necessary. Continue to cook until tofu is yellow and warm. Add in frozen vegetables or greens and cook until vegetables are warm or greens have softened. Add black salt (adds an eggy taste), hot sauce, and salsa if desired, plus salt and pepper to taste if desired.

Chef's Note Anything goes! But here are some of my favorite combos: sweet potato-black bean-spinach (with or without salsa), mushrooms and pizza sauce, spinach and black olives, tomatoes and spinach, black beans-corn-tomatoes, black beans-kale-sweet potato, black beans-kale-corn, sweet potatoes-hot sauce, and roasted potatoes with fresh chives. I also slip kale, bell peppers, or fresh dill in the scramble from time to time!

PER SERVING

Calories	219
Fat	10.2g
Carbs	13.3g
Fiber	6.3g
Sugars	2.1g
Protein	25.1g
WW Points	6

SERVES 2

15 oz firm tofu
3 tbsp nutritional yeast
1 tbsp Dijon mustard
1 tsp onion powder
1 tsp garlic powder
½ tsp ground cumin
¼ tsp turmeric
vegetables, greens, etc. (optional)
black salt (optional)
hot sauce (optional)
salsa (optional)

tempeh bacon

This tempeh bacon beats the pants off any store-bought veggie bacon you can find (if I do say so myself). It's a great side at breakfast or brunch, but it also makes for a mean BLT. Plus, at only 36 calories a slice (with no worry of saturated fats, either), you can load up!

PER SLICE

Calories 36
Fat 1.6g
Carbs 2.8g
Fiber 0g
Sugars 0.9g
Protein 3.1g
WW Points 1

MAKES ABOUT 15 SLICES

1 8-oz pkg tempeh

3–4 tbsp low-sodium soy sauce or gluten-free tamari

1 tbsp pure maple syrup

1–2 tbsp vegetable broth

1 tbsp apple cider vinegar

2 tsp liquid smoke

½ tsp garlic powder

¼ tsp onion powder

¼ tsp smoked paprika

Chef's Note Use the full 4 tbsp (¼ cup) of soy sauce or tamari if you like your "bacon" salty, but reduce broth to 1 tbsp.

Slice tempeh very thin longways (yielding 14–18 slices) and place in a 9x13 glass casserole dish, with no overlap, and set aside. In a small bowl, whisk all ingredients (except tempeh) together and pour over tempeh. Let tempeh marinate for four hours, flipping the strips over halfway through (after two hours), if possible. (Marinate until the tempeh has become brown and most of the marinade liquid has absorbed.) Heat oven to 300°F. Line a cookie sheet with parchment paper and place bacon strips on pre-pared cookie sheet, taking care to ensure no overlap. Bake for 10 minutes. Flip over and bake 5–10 more minutes or until tempeh is dark brown, crispy, and slightly charred on a few edges.

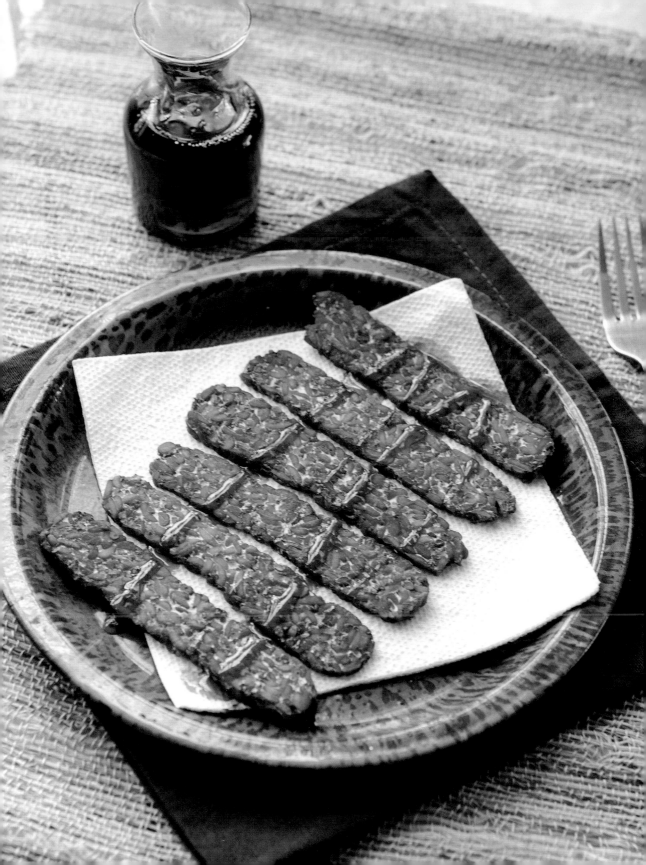

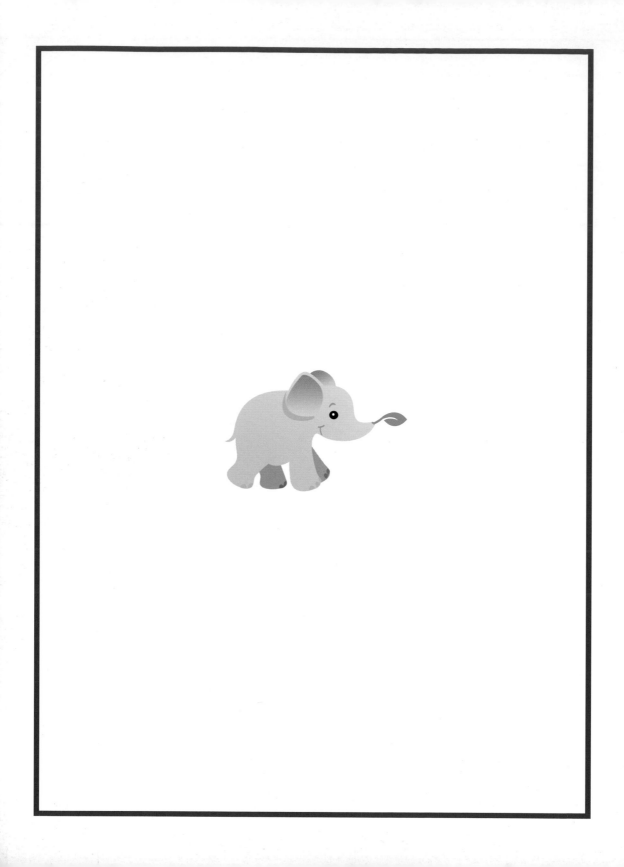

muffins & breads

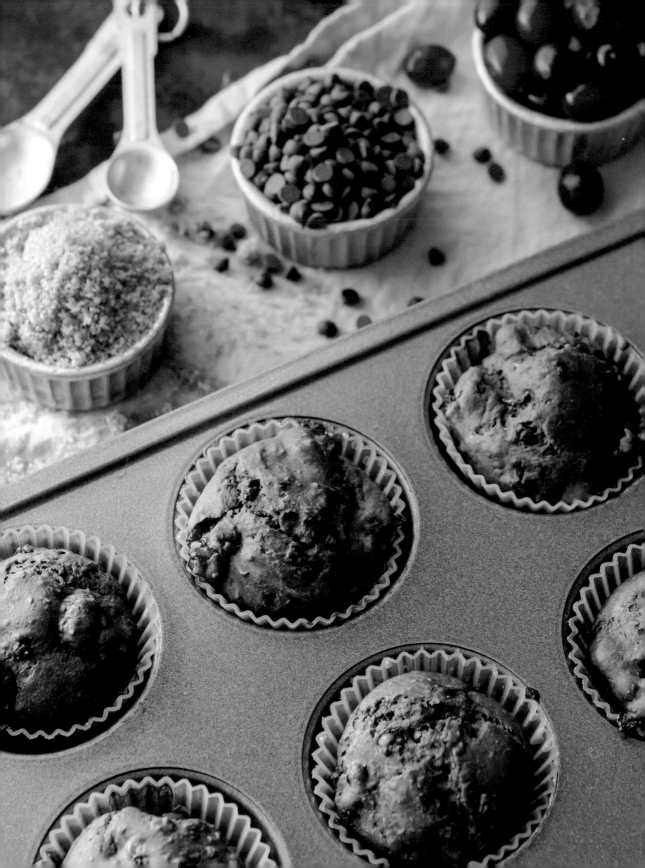

ruby chocolate muffins

Fresh cranberries are the "rubies" in this muffin. It's amazing what a little tartness does to a chocolate chip muffin. Seriously, who knew chocolate and cranberry go so well together? PS: These are perfect for potlucks during the holidays!

Preheat oven to 350°F. Line muffin tin with paper or silicone cups or use a nonstick pan, and set aside. In a mixing bowl, whisk flour, cocoa, baking powder, and sugar together. Add applesauce and nondairy milk, and stir until just combined. Stir in chocolate chips and cranberries, plus extract (if using). Spoon into prepared muffin tin and bake 15–20 minutes, until the muffins are firm to the touch and a toothpick inserted in the center comes out clean.

PER MUFFIN

Calories	105
Fat	1.9g
Carbs	21.1g
Fiber	3g
Sugars	6.7g
Protein	3.1g
WW Points	3

MAKES 12

- 1¾ c white whole-wheat flour
- ¼ c unsweetened cocoa
- 1 tbsp baking powder
- ¼– ½ c brown sugar
- ½ c unsweetened applesauce
- 1 c nondairy milk (plain or chocolate)
- ¼–½ c vegan chocolate chips
- 1 c fresh cranberries
- 1 tsp chocolate extract (optional)

Muffins are a great snack, dessert, and portable breakfast option for the busy health seeker who's always on the go.

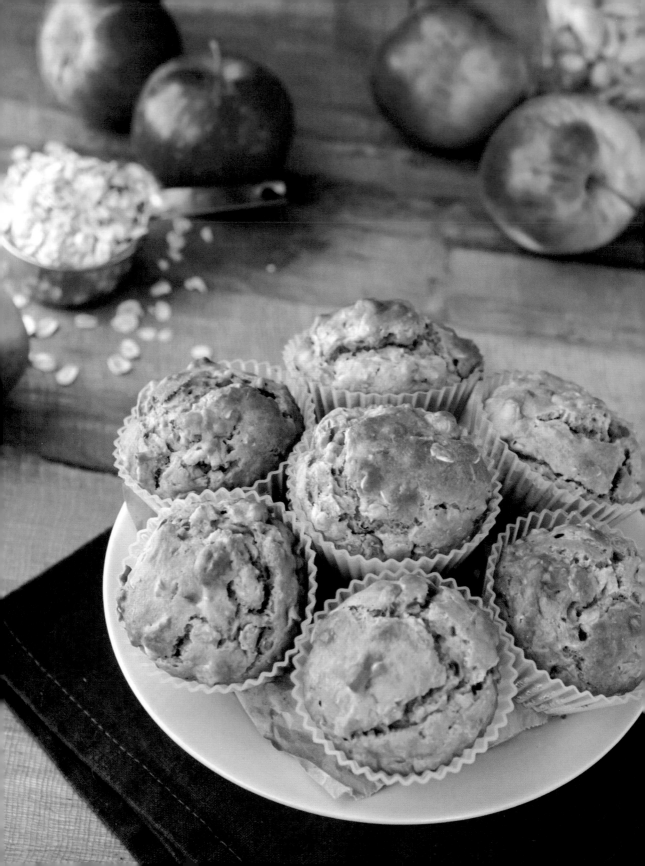

YUM! 9/14

✔ SOY-FREE ✔ QUICK ✔ BUDGET

"cheater" peanut butter muffins

These muffins are full of fresh fruit and oat goodness. I call them "cheater" muffins since I use a little bit of peanut butter in the recipe—but oh, how the flavor is worth it!

Preheat oven to 350°F. Line muffin tin with paper or silicone cups or use a nonstick pan, and set aside. Core and dice apple, measuring out 1 cup and placing the rest in a food processor or blender. In a mixing bowl, whisk flour, oats, baking powder, and baking soda together. Add diced apple and set aside. In the blender, add maple syrup or agave nectar, vanilla, water, nondairy milk, and banana, and whiz until smooth. Pour banana mixture into flour-apple mixture and stir a few times until mostly combined. Add peanut butter and stir until just combined. If the batter looks too dry (depends on the apple's juiciness), add a little more nondairy milk. Spoon into muffin pan and bake 15–20 minutes.

PER MUFFIN

Calories	99
Fat	1.8g
Carbs	19.1g
Fiber	2.1g
Sugars	7.4g
Protein	2.6g
WW Points	3

MAKES 12

- 1 red apple
- 1 c white whole-wheat flour
- ½ c rolled oats
- 2 tsp baking powder
- 1 tsp baking soda
- ¼ c pure maple syrup or agave nectar
- 2 tsp vanilla extract
- ¼ c water
- 2 tbsp nondairy milk
- 1 ripe banana
- 2 tbsp smooth peanut butter

PER MUFFIN

Calories 135
Fat. 2.5g
Carbs 25.4g
Fiber 1.4g
Sugars. 8.2g
Protein 2.7g
WW Points. 4

MAKES 12

- 1¾ c white whole-wheat flour
- 1 tbsp baking powder
- 2 tbsp brown sugar
- pinch salt (optional)
- ½ c nondairy milk (plain or vanilla), divided
- 2 very ripe bananas
- 1 tbsp vanilla extract
- ¼ c unsweetened applesauce
- ½ c vegan chocolate chips

Chef's Note Your bananas should be very ripe: spotted and with a strong banana smell.

chocolate chip muffins

Everyone's favorite cookie turned into a muffin! What I love most about these muffins is that they use hardly any sugar at all. Instead, the sweetness comes from bananas.

Preheat oven to 350°F. Line muffin tin with paper or silicone cups or use a nonstick pan, and set aside. In a mixing bowl, whisk flour, baking powder, and sugar together. In a food processor or blender, combine ¼ cup nondairy milk with bananas and vanilla extract until smooth. Then pour into flour mixture. Stir a few times, add applesauce and remaining ¼ cup milk, and stir until mostly combined. Gently fold in chips, stirring until just combined. Bake 15–20 minutes or until the muffins are golden, firm to the touch, and a toothpick inserted in the center comes out clean.

lemon-zucchini muffins

PER MUFFIN

Calories 81
Fat. 0.6g
Carbs 18.1g
Fiber 2.2g
Sugars. 5.2g
Protein 2.4g
WW Points 2

Firing up the hot oven is not my favorite thing to do in the summer, but it's totally worth it to make these light muffins using your garden-fresh zucchini! Plus you can totally fool your friends and kids into eating vegetables with these muffins!

Preheat oven to 350°F. Line muffin tin with paper or silicone cups or use a nonstick pan, and set aside. In a mixing bowl, whisk flour, baking powder, and salt together until well combined. In a blender or food processor, blend banana with ¼ cup nondairy milk until combined. Pour into flour mixture, then add remaining nondairy milk, yogurt, lemon zest, and extract (if using), and stir a few times. Add zucchini and sugar, and then stir until just combined. Spoon into muffin tin and bake 18–25 minutes.

MAKES 12

- 1½ c white whole-wheat flour
- 1 tbsp baking powder
- pinch salt
- 1 small, very ripe banana
- ¾ c nondairy milk (plain or vanilla), divided
- ½ c vegan yogurt (plain, lemon, or vanilla)
- zest of two small lemons
- 1–2 tsp lemon extract (optional)
- 1 c shredded zucchini
- ¼ c light brown sugar

Chef's Notes

» Use a cheese grater to shred zucchini. If your zucchini is really wet, try resting it on a clean kitchen towel or paper towel for a few minutes to absorb some of the excess moisture.

» These muffins are very lightly sweetened. For a sweeter muffin, bump the sugar up to ⅓ or ½ cup.

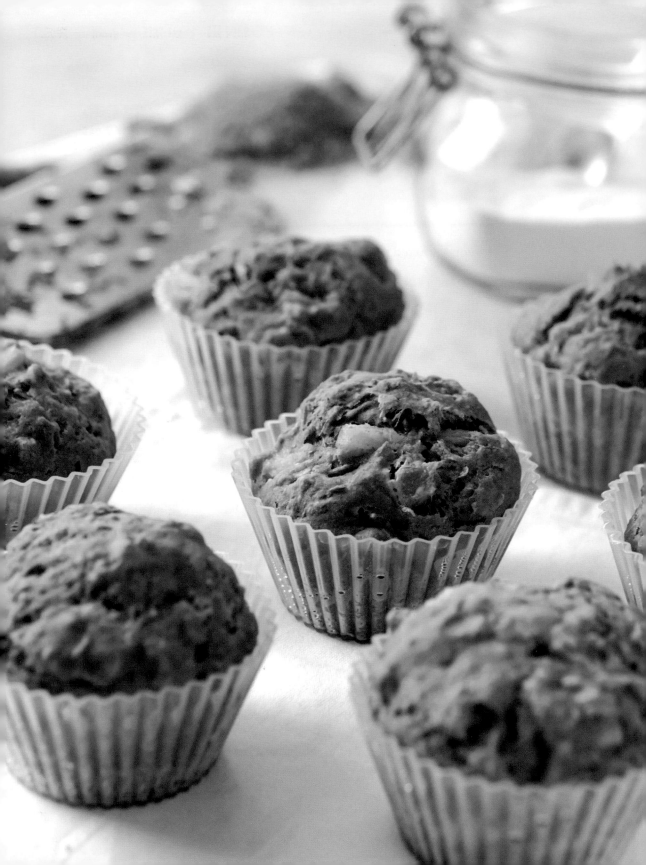

pineapple-carrot muffins

Knowing many traditional carrot cake recipes use pineapple for flavor, I started to wonder if I could make my Carrot Cake Cupcakes (from *The Happy Herbivore Cookbook*) into sugar-free muffins by using pineapple as a sweetener. I find you still need to use a little bit of sugar in this recipe, but otherwise, a low-sugar muffin (packed with fruits and vegetables!) has never tasted so good! These muffins are moist, lightly sweet, and incredibly filling.

Preheat oven to 350°F. Line muffin tin with paper or silicone cups or use a nonstick pan, and set aside. In a mixing bowl, whisk flour, baking soda, baking powder, ground cinnamon, and sugar together. Then stir in carrot, vanilla, pineapple juice, crushed pineapple, and applesauce (if using). If your batter seems dry, add another 1 tbsp of pineapple juice. Bake 15–25 minutes, until the muffins are firm to the touch and a toothpick inserted in the center comes out clean.

PER MUFFIN

Calories 72
Fat. 0.3g
Carbs 15.9g
Fiber 1.9g
Sugars. 4.5g
Protein 2.2g
WW Points 2

MAKES 12

- 1½ c white whole-wheat flour
- 1 tsp baking soda
- 1 tsp baking powder
- 1¼ tsp ground cinnamon
- 2 tbsp brown sugar
- 1 carrot, shredded
- 2 tsp vanilla extract
- ⅔ c pineapple juice (from can)
- ⅔ c crushed pineapple
- 2 tbsp applesauce (optional, for a very moist cake)

Chef's Note I don't bother to skin my carrot in this recipe. Also, if you only have diced pineapple, you can just chop it up with a knife.

UNDER 150 CALORIES

PER MUFFIN

Calories 116
Fat. 0.8g
Carbs 25.6g
Fiber 2.9g
Sugars. 8.8g
Protein 3.5g
WW Points 3

MAKES 12

- 2 c white whole-wheat flour
- 1 tsp baking powder
- ½ tsp baking soda
- pinch salt
- ¼ c raw sugar
- 1 ripe (spotted) banana
- ½ c vanilla nondairy milk, divided
- 6 oz vegan yogurt (plain, vanilla, or blueberry)
- ¼ c unsweetened applesauce
- 1 c blueberries (thawed, if using frozen)
- 3–4 tbsp lemon zest

blueberry yogurt muffins

If I had to pick a favorite kind of muffin, I think blueberry muffins would be it for me. With their hint of lemon, these muffins make me think of sunny, relaxed mornings. I also love that they're made with vegan yogurt (a boost of protein!) and very little sugar.

Preheat oven to 350°F. Line muffin tin with paper or silicone cups or use a nonstick pan, and set aside. In a mixing bowl, whisk flour with baking powder, baking soda, salt, and sugar. In a small food processor or blender, whiz banana with ¼ cup nondairy milk until silky smooth. Stir into flour mixture, then add yogurt, applesauce, and remaining nondairy milk. Stir a few times, add blueberries and lemon zest, and stir gently, folding in blueberries, until just combined. Spoon into muffin cups and bake 15–20 minutes or until muffins are golden, firm to the touch, and a toothpick inserted in the center comes out clean.

If you just want to make a single muffin, see Blueberry Muffin on page 50.

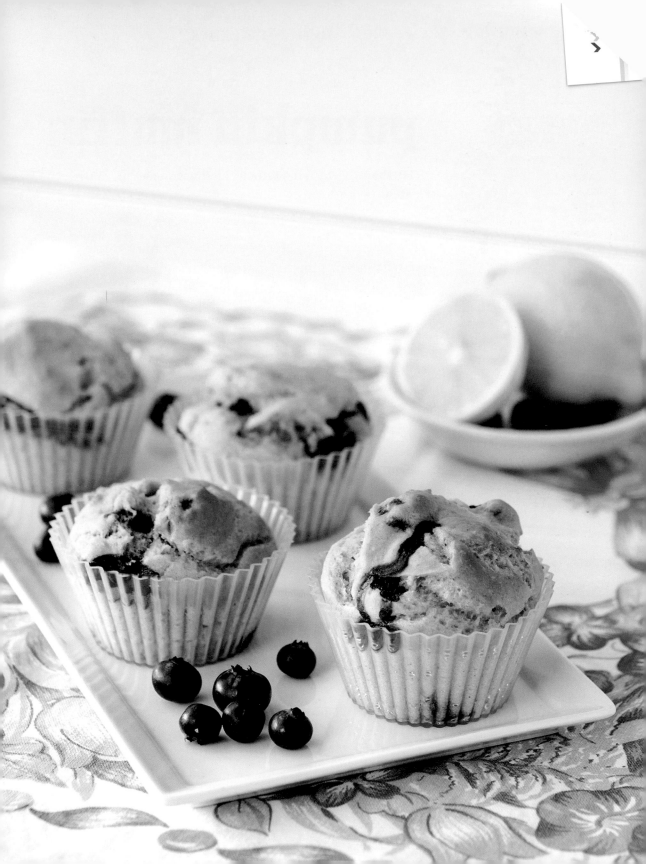

PER MUFFIN
PUMPKIN / BLUEBERRY

Calories	189/193
Fat	0.6g/0.5g
Carbs	44.3g/46.3g
Fiber	2.2g/1.1g
Sugars	21.7g/27.1g
Protein	2.9g/2.6g
WW Points	5/5

SINGLE SERVING

- 3 tbsp white whole-wheat flour
- ¼ tsp baking powder
- ½ tsp pumpkin pie spice
- 1 tbsp brown sugar
- 2 tbsp pure pumpkin (canned)
- 1 tbsp pure maple syrup
- 1 tbsp nondairy milk

SINGLE SERVING

- 3 tbsp white whole-wheat flour
- 2 tsp raw sugar
- 1 tbsp agave nectar or pure maple syrup
- 1 tbsp nondairy milk
- ¼ tsp baking powder
- 1½ tbsp blueberries (wild ones work best)
- pinch lemon zest (optional)

pumpkin muffin

Get the taste of fall—without having to bake an entire batch.

Preheat oven or toaster oven to 350°F. Line a single muffin cup or a metal 1-cup measuring cup with a liner, or use a foil baking cup (e.g., Reynolds) that will stand on its own or silicone cup, and set aside. In a small bowl, whisk dry ingredients together and then add remaining wet ingredients. Stir until combined, adding a little extra nondairy milk if necessary. Gently spoon into muffin cup and bake 15–18 minutes, until the muffin is firm to the touch and a toothpick inserted in the center comes out clean.

blueberry muffin

I love this muffin from *Everyday Happy Herbivore* so much that I had to include it here with some adjustments to make it (slightly) lower in calories.

Preheat oven or toaster oven to 350°F. Line a single muffin cup or a metal 1-cup measuring cup with a liner, or use a foil baking cup (e.g., Reynolds) that will stand on its own or silicone cup, and set aside. Add all ingredients in order in small mixing bowl, and then stir until completely combined. Transfer batter to muffin cup and bake 15–20 minutes or until a toothpick inserted in the center comes out clean.

breakfast corn muffins

These corn muffins are lightly sweet and have the added bonus of carrots. Good morning indeed!

Preheat oven to 350°F. Line muffin tin with paper or silicone cups or use a nonstick pan, and set aside. In a mixing bowl, whisk cornmeal, flour, baking powder, and salt together. Add remaining ingredients in order and stir to combine. Bake 15–20 minutes, until the muffins are firm to the touch and a toothpick inserted in the center comes out clean.

Chef's Note You can also add 1 cup corn, if you like, but you will probably yield an extra muffin or two. If your corn is frozen, expect bake time to increase by a few minutes.

PER MUFFIN
(WITHOUT ADDED SUGAR)

Calories 101
Fat. 0.8g
Carbs 21.9g
Fiber 1.4g
Sugars. 4.5g
Protein 2.1g
WW Points 3

MAKES 12

- 1 c yellow cornmeal
- 1 c white whole-wheat flour
- 1 tbsp baking powder
  pinch salt (¼ tsp optional)
  2 carrots, minced or finely chopped
- 1 c nondairy milk
- ¼ c pure maple syrup or agave nectar
- 1–1½ tsp lemon zest (zest of small lemon)
- 2 tbsp raw sugar (optional)

PER BISCUIT
(WITHOUT GLAZE)

Calories 125
Fat 2.7g
Carbs 23.5g
Fiber 2.8g
Sugars 6.7g
Protein 3.5g
WW Points 3

MAKES 6

1 c white whole-wheat flour

2 tsp baking powder

pinch salt

1 spotted banana

¼–½ c nondairy milk

¼ c vegan chocolate chips, or more if you love chocolate!

Chef's Notes

» Raisins also work great instead of chocolate chips.

» You can mix powdered sugar with a little nondairy milk and a drop or two of almond or vanilla extract to make a glaze/icing, too!

banana-chocolate chip scones

Okay, so these are really drop biscuits, but they like to pretend to be scones, and we don't want to take that away from them, do we? They are so, so good!

Preheat oven to 400°F. Line a cookie sheet with parchment paper and set aside. Whisk flour, baking powder, and salt together in a mixing bowl. Break banana in half and add both halves to the flour, and then start mixing it together with your hands, squishing the banana through your fingers. Keep mixing the banana into the flour until you have a bowl of flour balls. Add ¼ cup nondairy milk and chocolate chips, and stir to combine, adding more milk if necessary (when in doubt, wetter is better). Drop six similar-sized spoonfuls on prepared cookie sheet and bake 10–12 minutes, until the scones are firm and golden at the edges.

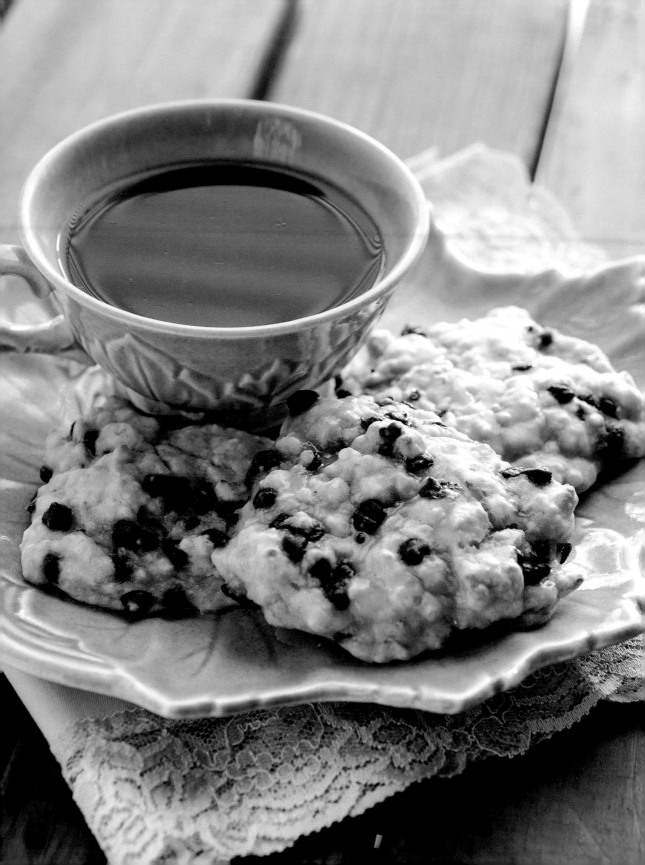

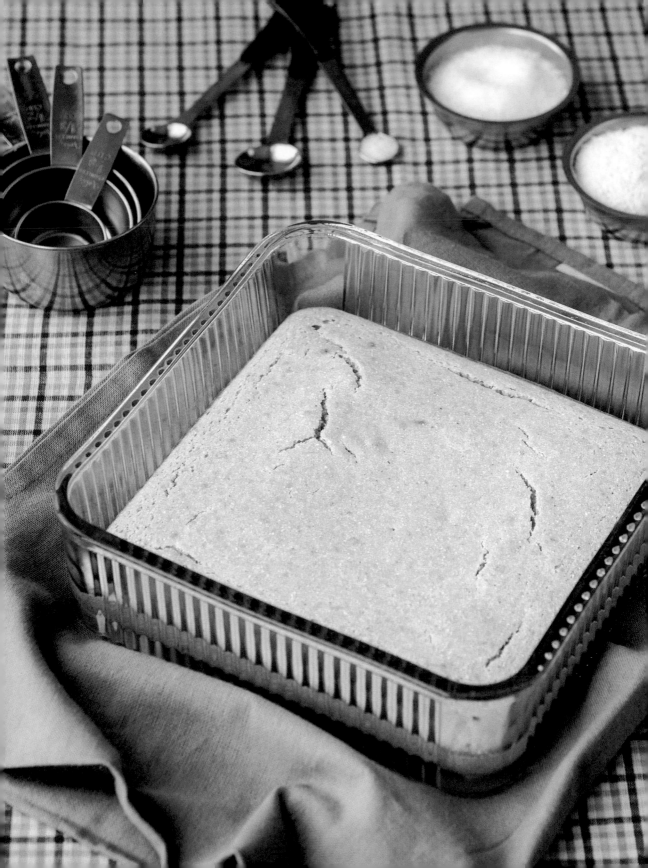

classic cornbread

You may recognize this cornbread recipe from my previous cookbooks (it's always making the rounds). It's a favorite and for good reason: You need only a handful of pantry staples to make it happen, it's foolproof, and you can adapt it to fit the occasion. Add some jalapeños for a hot-n-spicy cornbread. Add diced bell peppers for a fiesta-style cornbread. Add sweet frozen corn kernels or roasted corn kernels with a dash of smoked paprika, and so on. I even once added pumpkin when I was out of applesauce, and that was awesome. Plus, all the fiber from the flour and cornmeal makes one slice very filling.

Preheat oven to 400°F and set aside a 9-inch glass dish or nonstick square baking pan (I also love a springform pan for this recipe). In a mixing bowl, whisk cornmeal, flour, and baking powder together. Add nondairy milk, applesauce, maple syrup or agave nectar, and sugar if using. Stir a few times, add in optional ingredients if using, and then stir until just combined. Pour batter into pan and bake approximately 20 minutes—you want it to be golden, starting to crack, and firm to the touch. When a toothpick is inserted in the center, it should come out clean.

PER SERVING

Calories 131
Fat. 1g
Carbs 28.7g
Fiber 1.6g
Sugars. 6g
Protein 2.6g
WW Points 3

SERVES 9

- 1 c yellow cornmeal
- 1 c white whole-wheat flour
- 1 tbsp baking powder
- 1 c nondairy milk
- ¼ c unsweetened applesauce
- ¼ c pure maple syrup or agave nectar
- 2 tbsp raw sugar (optional)

Chef's Note You can replace 2 tbsp of the maple syrup with 2–3 tbsp additional nondairy milk for a less sweet cornbread.

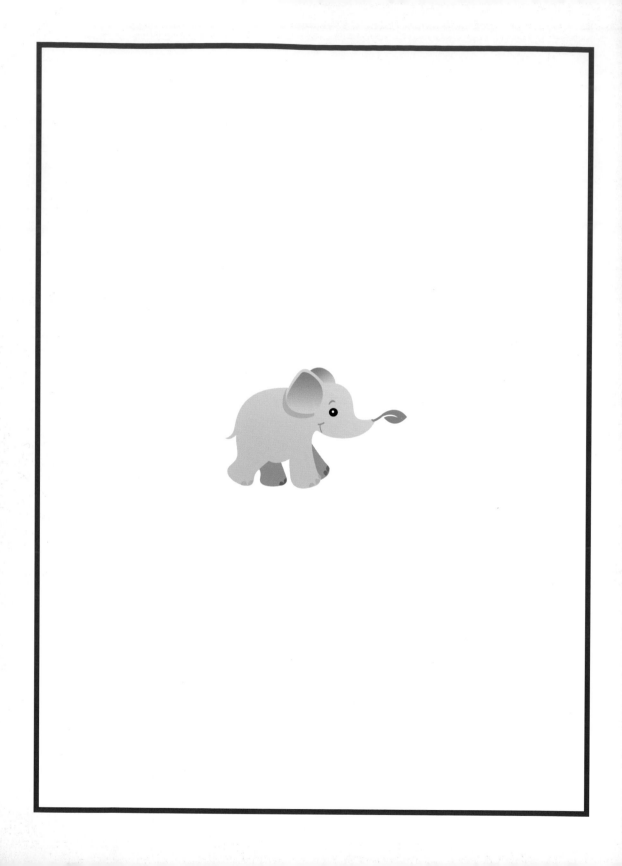

sandwiches, tacos & more

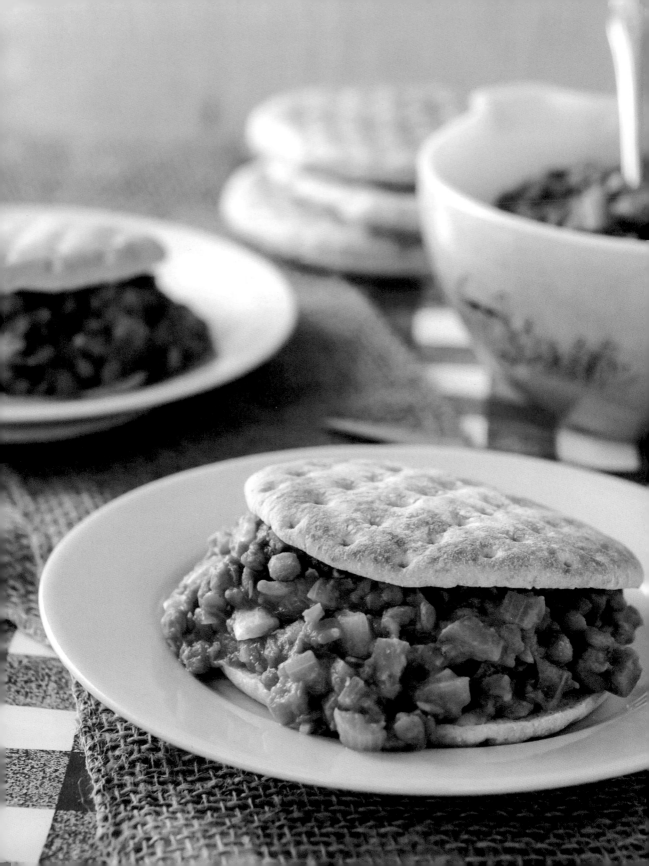

lentil joes

Sloppy joes—or, as my family calls them, "wimpies"—were one of my favorite childhood foods before I became a vegetarian. I've never had much success mimicking my mom's recipe (vegan or not—I swear she's holding back a secret ingredient!), so I decided to take a totally new approach and use lentils. It's not Mom's meatloaf-er, sloppy joes—but this recipe is deliciously different, quite filling, and very easy to make!

Line a large skillet with a thin layer of vegetable broth and sauté onion, garlic, and bell peppers until onion is translucent, bell peppers have softened and turned a mellow green, and most of the broth has evaporated. Add remaining ingredients (hot sauce or cayenne as desired, plus a few dashes of smoked paprika) and stir to combine. Warm, stirring occasionally, over low, and then serve.

For years my lunchbox revolved around a sandwich. Although I've become more creative with my lunches over the past few plant-based years, I still love going back to the classic sandwich with two sides option.

PER SERVING
(ABOUT ½ CUP)

Calories	131
Fat	0.7g
Carbs	23.9g
Fiber	7.8g
Sugars	6.7g
Protein	8.7g
WW Points	3

MAKES 6

- vegetable broth
- 1 onion, diced
- 2 garlic cloves, minced
- 1 green bell pepper, seeded and diced
- ½ c tomato sauce
- 2 tbsp ketchup
- 1 tbsp prepared yellow mustard
- 1 tbsp Dijon mustard
- 1 tbsp low-sodium soy sauce or gluten-free tamari
- 1 tsp Vegan Worcestershire Sauce (pg. 266) (optional)
- 2½ c cooked lentils
- ¼ tsp ground cumin
- 1–2 tbsp brown sugar
- hot sauce or cayenne pepper
- smoked paprika

PER SERVING
(ABOUT ½ CUP)

Calories 79
Fat 2.7g
Carbs 10.1g
Fiber 1.9g
Sugars 6.9g
Protein 5.8g
WW Points 2

SERVES 5

8 oz (1¾ c) extra-firm tofu, diced

2 celery stalks, sliced or diced

1 c red grapes, sliced in half

1 c green grapes, sliced in half

2–3 tbsp Vegan Mayo (pg. 262)

2 tbsp nutritional yeast

1 tsp Italian seasoning or Poultry Seasoning Mix (pg. 268)

¼ tsp garlic powder

½ tsp onion powder

black pepper, to taste

pecans or candied pecans or walnuts or slivered almonds (optional)

sonoma "chicken" salad

They just do chicken salad differently in California! I didn't grow up eating chicken salad; it was introduced to me at college—canned chicken, relish, mayo, celery, and mustard mixed together—and that's all I knew until I moved to California. I was plant-based by then, but I was surprised to see chicken salad sold in the deli mixed with grapes and nuts. I learned this variation is attributed to Sonoma Valley (wine country) and just had to make a version I could eat. I'm glad I did! Crisp, refreshing, and oh-so-satisfying, this salad is fine for a sandwich, out of the bowl with a spoon, or scooped on top of lettuce or spinach.

Combine all ingredients together. Taste, adding more black pepper, nutritional yeast, or Italian seasoning or poultry seasoning as needed.

Chef's Notes

» I find super protein tofu works best here.

» For an even more chicken-y flavor, sauté the tofu in ½ cup No-Chicken Broth (pg. 264) until the broth evaporates and tofu becomes golden. Allow tofu to cool before you make the salad.

» For a soy-free option, use a 15-oz can chickpeas, drained and rinsed (whole or mashed with a fork), instead of tofu and plain vegan yogurt (unsweetened if possible) instead of mayo. You might want to add a little bit of lemon juice to the yogurt to make it more mayo-like in flavor.

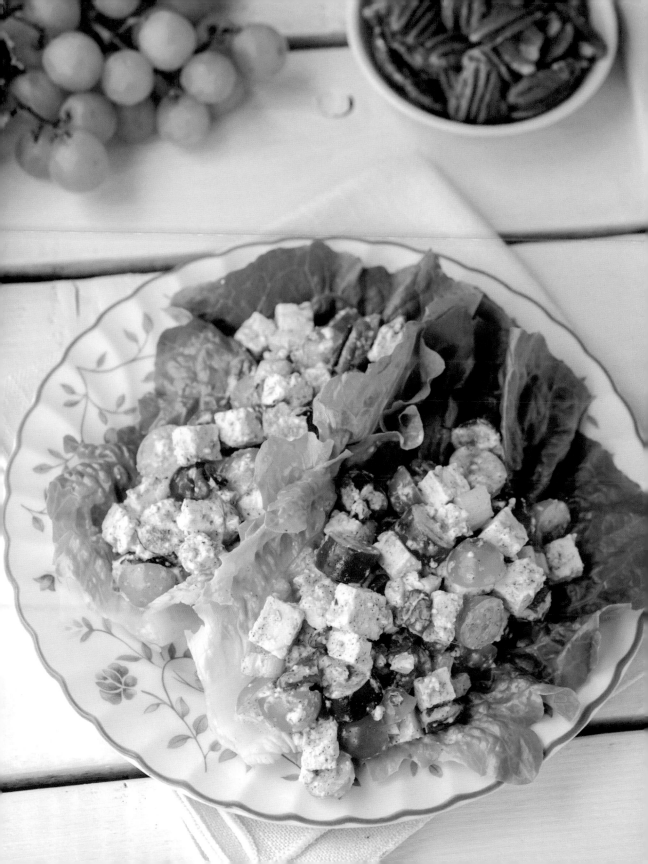

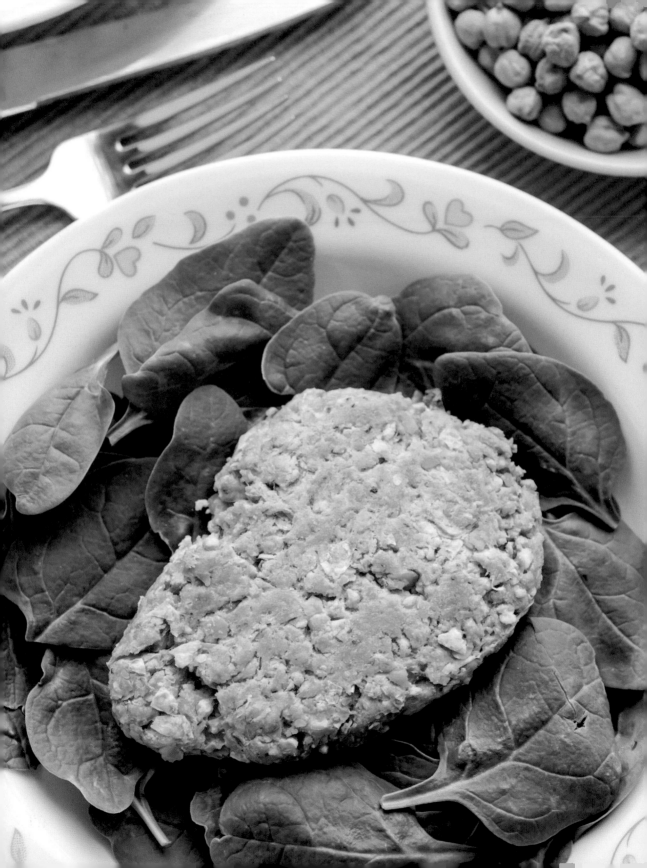

chickpea tenders

You might remember my chickpea tenders from *Every-day Happy Herbivore*. Here I've simplified my original recipe, but you still get deliciously filling and very versatile chickpea tenders! I use these for making "chicken" sandwiches, for dipping in barbecue sauce, and for topping my salad.

Preheat oven to 350°F. Line cookie sheet with parchment paper and set aside. In a mixing bowl, mash chickpeas with a fork until no whole beans are left. Add seasoning, nutritional yeast, Dijon, and hummus, and stir to combine. Add gluten and vegetable broth, then mix, using your hands, to form dough. Add more broth if you need to, but you don't want it too wet. Let rest for 5 minutes. Divide into four equal pieces. Roll each piece into a ball, then flatten out into a circle (like a chicken breast) with your palm. Bake for 10 minutes, flip them over, bake for 10 more minutes, flip them over again, and bake for 10 minutes. You can flip and bake a fourth time for 5–10 minutes if necessary. You want the tenders firm, crispy on the outside, and golden, but not overcooked, dried, or burnt on the edges.

PER TENDER

Calories	183
Fat	2.1g
Carbs	28.9g
Fiber	6.2g
Sugars	0g
Protein	13.7g
WW Points	4

MAKES 4

- 1 15-oz can chickpeas, drained and rinsed
- 1 tsp Poultry Seasoning Mix (pg. 268) or Italian seasoning
- 2 tbsp nutritional yeast
- 1½ tsp Dijon mustard
- 1 tbsp hummus
- 5 tbsp vital wheat gluten
- 3 tbsp low-sodium vegetable broth

Chef's Note You can substitute Vegan Mayo (pg. 262), vegan yogurt, or silken tofu for the hummus.

thai tacos

PER TACO

Calories 152
Fat 1.4g
Carbs 28.4g
Fiber 5.8g
Sugars 3.7g
Protein 6.1g
WW Points 4

My beloved chickpea tacos get reinvented with a little Thai flavoring and cool coleslaw. These tacos come together in a snap but present beautifully and are perfect in the summer when it's too hot to cook. The slaw is also great on its own as a side!

MAKES 6

1 15-oz can chickpeas, drained and rinsed

chili powder

4 c shredded cabbage (green, red, or a combination)

1 tbsp Vegan Mayo (pg. 262) or plain vegan yogurt

2–3 tbsp sweet red chili sauce, divided

lime zest

juice of 1 small lime

sea salt (optional)

1–2 green onions, sliced

Asian hot sauce (e.g., Sriracha; optional)

6 corn tortillas

cilantro (optional)

Mash chickpeas with a fork in a small bowl until they crumble. Sprinkle with chili powder as desired, stir, and sprinkle again to taste, then set aside. In another bowl, combine cabbage with mayo, 2 tbsp chili sauce, 1 tsp lime zest (about ½ of the small lime), and juice from 1 lime slice, and stir to combine. Taste, adding more chili sauce, lime juice, or zest as desired. I also like to add a pinch of sea salt. Stir in green onion, reserving some for garnish. (For a spicier dish, you can also add an Asian hot sauce like Sriracha to taste.) Spoon chickpea mixture into tortillas. Top with slaw. Garnish with a few green onions and cilantro leaves if using. Drizzle with extra hot sauce if desired (a little goes a long way; it's explosive!).

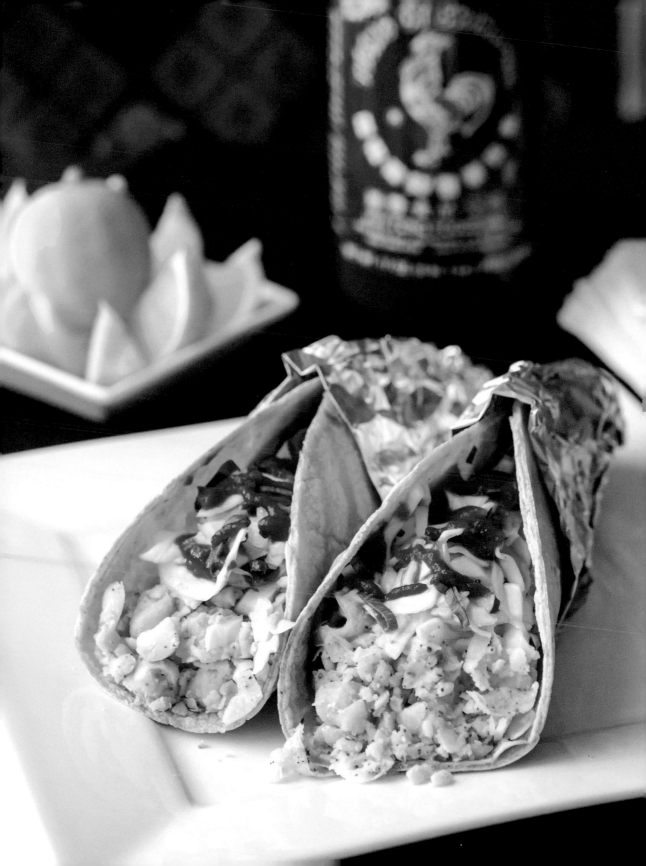

PER SERVING

Calories 193
Fat. 9.1g
Carbs 14.1g
Fiber 3.1g
Sugars. 5.4g
Protein 18.2g
WW Points. 5

SERVES 2

1 lb extra-firm tofu,
   pressed

Lime slices (garnish)

JERK SAUCE

3 green onions, sliced

1–2 tsp allspice

⅛ tsp ground cinnamon

2 tsp fresh thyme

1 tbsp apple cider
   vinegar

2 tbsp ketchup

½ –1 tsp liquid smoke

¼ c vegetable broth

1 tbsp cornstarch

dash ground nutmeg

jerk tofu

Jerk is a style of cooking native to Jamaica involving a dry rub or wet marinade. The main flavor in jerk seasoning is allspice, that little canister on your spice rack that's typically neglected unless you're doing a little holiday-themed baking. (Now you have a use for it!) Jerk flavoring is different than anything you've had before, but it's oh-so-delicious. I like to serve this tofu over rice with lime garnish.

Slice tofu into 8–10 cutlets and bake 10 minutes. Flip them over and bake another 10 minutes. Repeat as necessary until golden or cooked as you like (I like mine very golden and firm). Meanwhile, whisk all ingredients of sauce together. Heat over low so it thickens into a glaze but be careful not to boil. Toss sauce with baked tofu and serve with a lime wedge.

quinoa taco meat

Is it obvious we love tacos in my house? I love this whole-some taco meat on a salad or on nachos with my Quick Nacho Sauce (pg. 212), but it's also great in a corn tortilla to make a soft taco or even slipped into a burrito. Get all the healthy benefits of eating quinoa with a taste of tacos, too!

Combine all ingredients in saucepan and cover. Bring to a boil, reduce heat to low, and simmer until liquid has evaporated and quinoa is fluffy, about 15 minutes. Taste, adding more hot sauce or cayenne as desired.

PER SERVING
(¼ CUP)

Calories	55
Fat	1g
Carbs	9.3g
Fiber	1.7g
Sugars	0g
Protein	2.6g
WW Points	1

SERVES 7

- 1 c No-Beef Broth (pg. 264)
- ½ c uncooked quinoa
- 1 tbsp chili powder
- 1 tsp ground cumin
- ½ tsp paprika
- ¼ tsp onion powder
- ¼ tsp garlic powder
- ½ tsp dried oregano
- cayenne or hot sauce to taste

On the 7-Day Meal Plans, I like to add sides that don't feel like "sides" or snacks. For example, I love adding a baked potato with salsa, hummus on a slice of toast with a tomato, a steamed sweet potato with cinnamon, or steamed broccoli sprinkled with nutritional yeast or AJ's Vegan Parmesan (pg. 271). Tofu drizzled with teriyaki sauce is another satisfying fave!

PER PATTY

Calories	128
Fat	1.4g
Carbs	17.8g
Fiber	3.9g
Sugars	0.1g
Protein	9.9g
WW Points	2

MAKES 6

- 1 15-oz can white beans, drained and rinsed
- 3 tbsp vegan mayo (vegan yogurt, silken tofu, or hummus will also work)
- 2 tbsp Dijon mustard
- 1 tbsp nutritional yeast
- 1 tsp onion powder
- 1 tsp garlic powder
- 1½ tsp mild yellow curry powder
- 1 c cooked quinoa
- ⅓ c vital wheat gluten
- 2–3 tbsp vegetable broth

Chef's Note Any white beans, such as navy, cannellini, or butter bean, will work in this recipe.

quinoa curry cakes

I like to eat these cakes topped with a smidge of hummus or a dollop of vegan yogurt over a bed of steamed leafy greens (dressed with a little fresh lemon juice), but they're great in a sandwich, too.

Preheat oven to 450°F. Line a cookie sheet with parchment paper and set aside. Mash beans with a fork in a mixing bowl until they have the consistency of refried beans. Add remaining ingredients in order and stir to combine, adding broth as necessary. With wet hands, pick off one-sixth of the mixture, roll into a ball, flatten, and shape into a patty. Repeat until all of the mixture is used. You may need to rinse your hands every other patty to prevent sticking. Bake 8 minutes, flip the patties over and bake 8 more minutes, then flip them again and bake for 5 minutes, but only if necessary. When the burgers are firm—brown along the edges and crisp on the outside—they are done.

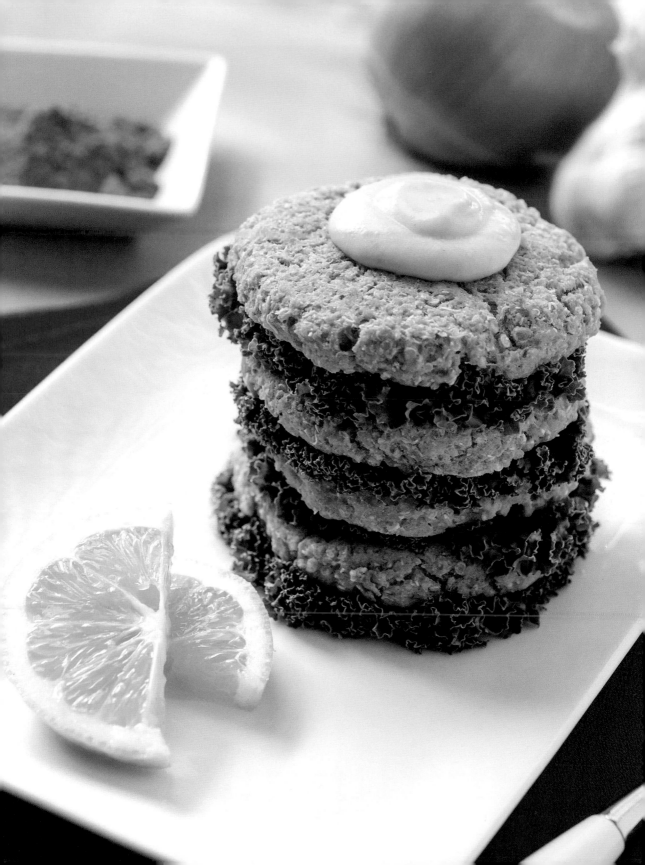

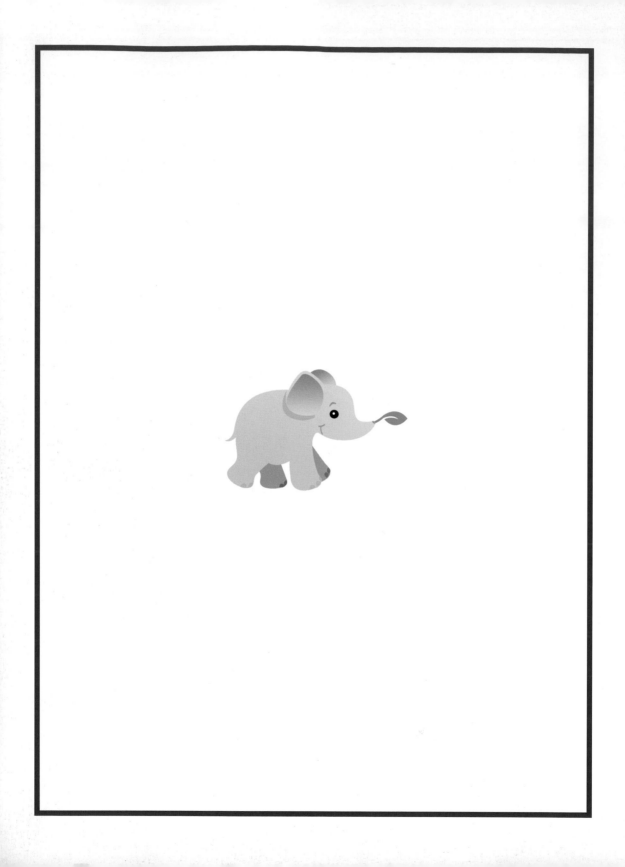

hearty burgers

✓ SOY-FREE ✓ GLUTEN-FREE ✓ QUICK ✓ BUDGET

UNDER 150 CALORIES

pesto burgers

PER PATTY

Calories 112
Fat. 1.4g
Carbs 18.5g
Fiber 5g
Sugars. 1.2g
Protein 7.1g
WW Points. 3

MAKES 4

- 1 15-oz can white beans, drained and rinsed
- ¼ –⅓ c minced fresh basil
- 1 tbsp nutritional yeast
- 1 tsp onion powder
- 1 tsp garlic powder
- ¼ tsp Italian seasoning
- 2½ tbsp Vegan Mayo (pg. 262) or plain vegan yogurt
- 1 tsp Dijon mustard
- ⅓ c instant oats

Chef's Note While any white bean (e.g., navy, butter bean, etc.) will do here, I prefer cannellini beans, also called white kidney beans.

Bean burgers go gourmet! (It's amazing what a little fresh basil can do for one's image.) I like to eat these burgers "straight up"—no bun, no nothin'—but they're great any way you wish to serve them and really filling. Sometimes I add a little Red Pesto (pg. 156) or marinara sauce on top.

Preheat oven to 400°F. Line a cookie sheet with parchment paper and set aside. In a mixing bowl, mash beans with a fork until mostly pureed but still some whole and half bean parts are left. Stir in basil (I send mine through a mini food processor), nutritional yeast, spices, and condiments, plus black pepper and salt if desired, stirring until well combined. Add oats and combine. Divide mixture into four equal portions and shape into patties. Bake patties for 10 minutes, flip them over, and bake for another 5–7 minutes, or until lightly crisp and golden on the outside.

pizza burgers

We tend to eat these burgers as patties topped with marinara and a sprinkle of AJ's Vegan Parmesan (pg. 271) instead of as a "burger" per se, but if you want to eat them burger-style, still add marinara, plus spinach and a slice of vegan mozzarella or dollop of Cream Sauce (pg. 157).

Preheat oven to 400°F. Line a cookie sheet with parchment paper and set aside. In a mixing bowl, mash beans with a fork until mostly pureed but still some whole and half bean parts are left. Stir in sauce and spices (a few dashes of Italian seasoning) until well combined. Then mix in oats. Divide into four equal portions and shape into thin patties. Bake for 10 minutes, flip the patties over, and bake another 5–7 minutes or until crusty on the outside and lightly golden.

PER PATTY

Calories	124
Fat	0.5g
Carbs	22.6g
Fiber	6.9g
Sugars	1g
Protein	7.1g
WW Points	3

MAKES 4

- 1 15-oz can white beans, drained and rinsed
- ¼ c pizza sauce or Marinara Sauce (pg. 263)
- 1 tsp onion powder
- 1 tsp garlic powder
- Italian seasoning
- ⅓ c instant oats

Chef's Note Any white bean such as navy, cannellini, etc. will work here.

Bean burgers are my solution for dinner any night I'm not in the mood to cook. Those nights come pretty often, and sometimes twice in a row, leaving my husband to say, "Burgers again?" I've gotten a little creative with my burgers, fusing cuisines in recipes like tacos and pizza.

taco burgers

Our favorite way to eat these burgers is slipped into a corn tortilla with corn shaved fresh off the cob, topped with ketchup or salsa and guacamole. *Arriba! Arriba!*

Preheat oven to 400°F. Line a cookie sheet with parchment paper and set aside. In a mixing bowl, mash beans with a fork until mostly pureed but still some half beans and bean parts are left. Stir in seasoning, ketchup, mustard, and mayo, and stir until well combined, then mix in oats. Divide mixture into eight equal portions and shape into patties. (They might feel a little wet, but they're fine. Rinse off your hands frequently while shaping the patties.) Bake patties for 10 minutes, flip them over, and bake for another 5–7 minutes or until lightly crusty on the outside. Slap into a bun or tortilla with choice toppings.

Chef's Note As a warning, some taco mixes are super hot or really salty. I suggest tasting yours first and if it's salty or explosive, add half to start. Taste the mixture and add more if desired.

PER PATTY

Calories 72
Fat 0.5g
Carbs 12.9g
Fiber 4.9g
Sugars 2.1g
Protein 4.5g
WW Points 2

MAKES 8

- 1 15-oz can black beans, drained and rinsed
- 1 15-oz can kidney beans, drained and rinsed
- 1 taco seasoning packet
- ¼ c ketchup or tomato sauce
- 2 tbsp prepared yellow mustard
- 2 tbsp Vegan Mayo (pg. 262) or plain vegan yogurt
- ⅔ c instant oats
- 8 buns or corn tortillas
- toppings

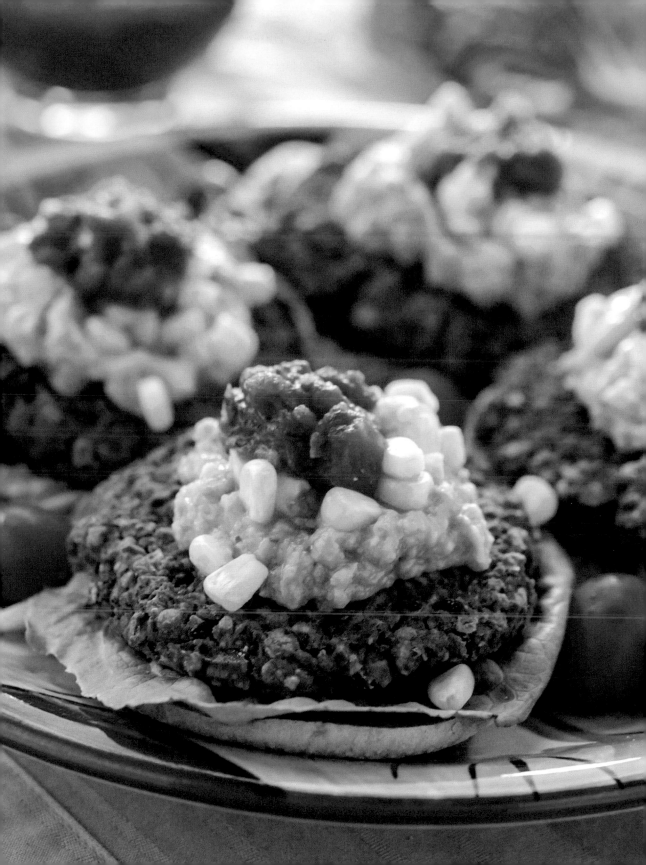

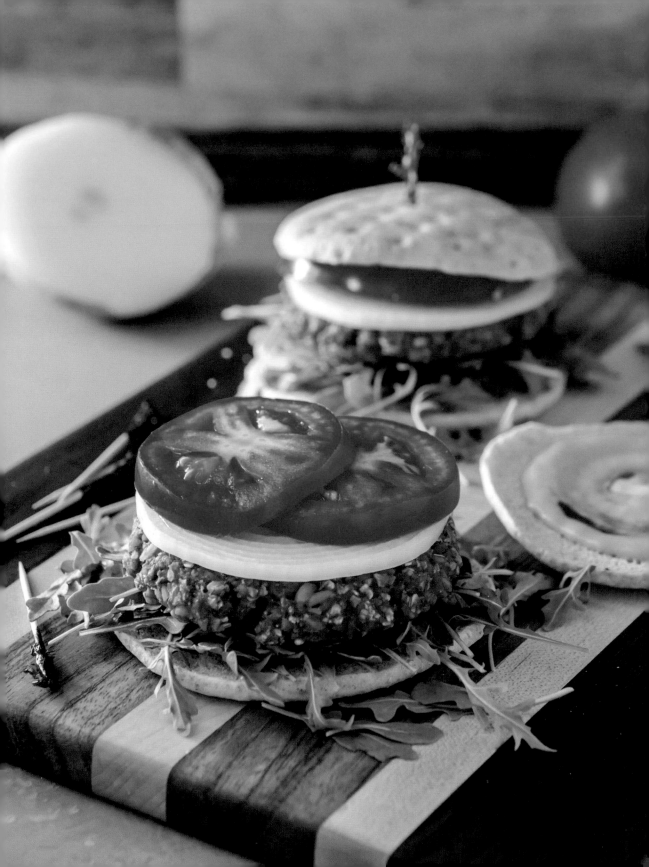

tempeh burgers

I tend to favor beans when making vegetarian burgers but thought I'd give tempeh a chance. Delicious! I love the nutty flavor the tempeh lends to this burger and it's a great "basic" burger that lets all the toppings shine. If you're new to meatless burgers, this is a good place to start!

Preheat oven to 350°F. Line cookie sheet with parchment paper and set aside. Shred tempeh using a cheese grater so it's crumbled. Transfer crumbled tempeh to a mixing bowl and add ketchup, mustard, barbecue sauce, soy sauce or tamari, onion powder, garlic powder, Italian seasoning, Worcestershire sauce, and 8–10 dashes each of curry powder and ground cumin. Using a spatula, stir to combine, and then add instant oats and stir to combine again. Add vital wheat gluten and 2 tbsp broth, and stir to combine. Add more broth as necessary so it's wet and combining and there is no visible flour dusting. Break into six equal amounts and shape into patties. Bake 10 minutes, flip the patties over, and bake another 5–7 minutes until as crisp and firm as you like, noting that they firm a bit as they cool.

PER BURGER

Calories 169
Fat 7.2g
Carbs 15.2g
Fiber 1.4g
Sugars 4.8g
Protein 13.2g
WW Points 3

MAKES 6

8 oz tempeh
3 tbsp ketchup
3 tbsp mustard
3 tbsp barbecue sauce
1 tbsp low-sodium soy sauce or gluten-free tamari
1 tsp onion powder
1 tsp garlic powder
1½ tbsp Italian seasoning
1 tsp Vegan Worcestershire Sauce (pg. 266)
mild yellow curry powder
ground cumin
½ c instant oats
5 tbsp vital wheat gluten
2–4 tbsp vegetable broth

Chef's Note If you want your patties rather dark brown, add ¼ tsp browning sauce.

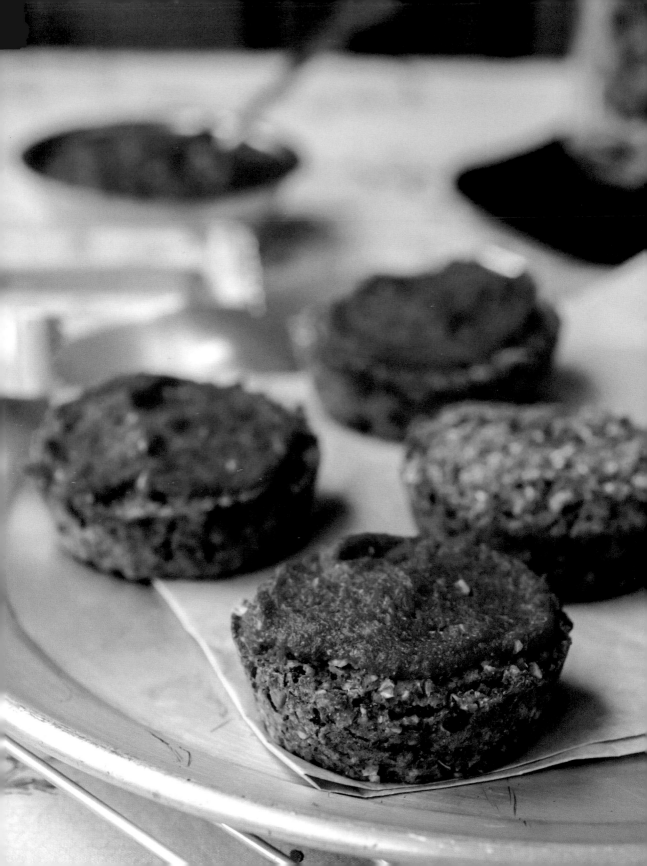

meatloaf bites

One afternoon I grabbed what I thought was corn from the freezer but later realized it was mixed vegetables. Once they thawed on the counter I knew they weren't going back in, so I looked for a new, inventive way to use them. A can of kidney beans started calling, and before I knew it I had a vegetable-filled meatloaf in the oven. Since this meatloaf is baked in a muffin tin (great for serving sizes and portion control), I call it meatloaf "bites" and, yes, leftovers are great as a burger!

Preheat oven to 350°F. Line a muffin tin with paper liners or use nonstick. Mash beans in a bowl with fork or potato masher until well mashed. Add remaining ingredients, except oats, and stir to combine. Stir in oats. Spoon into muffin tin and pack down. Bake for 20 minutes until crisp on the outside and fairly firm to the touch (firms a bit as it cools). Serve with ketchup, Quick Gravy (pg. 188), etc.

PER BITE

Calories	101
Fat	1.7g
Carbs	16.9g
Fiber	6.5g
Sugars	3g
Protein	5.8g
WW Points	2

MAKES 8

- 1 15-oz can kidney beans, drained and rinsed
- 1 tbsp onion powder
- 1 tbsp garlic powder
- 1 tbsp Italian seasoning
- 1 tbsp chili powder (add another 1 tsp if you like it spicy)
- 3 tbsp ketchup
- 2 tbsp mustard
- 1 tbsp Vegan Worcestershire Sauce (pg. 266)
- 1 c frozen mixed vegetables, thawed
- 6 tbsp instant oats

Chef's Note Pipe Easy Mashed Potatoes (pg. 187) on top.

lentil & oat burgers

Beans take a back seat with these filling lentil and oat burgers. I tend to serve these more as patties with a sauce on top rather than as a traditional burger, but you can do what you like. Lentils, by the way, are a bit dryer than beans, so be careful not to overbake, and you probably want to have something creamy on the burger—like Vegan Mayo (pg. 262), or my lemon crème (below), too.

PER PATTY

Calories	115
Fat	1.1g
Carbs	20.1g
Fiber	7.3g
Sugars	2.3g
Protein	3.8g
WW Points	2

MAKES 6

- 2 c cooked lentils
- 1½ tsp Vegan Worcestershire Sauce (pg. 266)
- 3 tbsp Dijon mustard
- 2 tbsp ketchup
- 1 tsp onion powder
- 1 tsp garlic powder
- 1 tsp ground cumin
- 1½ tsp ground coriander
- ½ c rolled oats
- juice of 1 small lemon (about 2–3 tbsp)
- lemon zest (optional)

Chef's Note Add lemon zest to the burger batter for a stronger lemon flavoring.

Preheat oven to 350°F. Line a cookie sheet with parchment paper and set aside. Pulse lentils in a food processor or blender so most become chewed up and mush-like, but some whole and half lentils still remain. Transfer to a mixing bowl, add vegan Worcestershire sauce, mustard, ketchup, and spices, and stir to combine. Add oats and stir to combine. Add juice of a small lemon, stirring to combine one last time. Divide into six equal portions and shape into patties. Bake 10 minutes, flip the patties over, and bake another 5 minutes, or until firm and crisp on the outside, being careful not to overbake.

LEMON CRÈME

Combine plain vegan yogurt or mayo with a little lemon juice and lemon zest to taste. You can also add a dash of ground coriander.

A BURGER WITH THE WORKS!

Sometimes I love a bun (or a tortilla) and condiments with my burger to shake things up! Here are the caloric values for the "extras" so you can build your perfect burger.

ITEM	CALORIES
Corn tortilla (1)	52
Whole-wheat bun (1)	100–120
Lettuce (leaf)	1
Tomato (slice)	1
Onion (slice)	1
Guacamole (regular; 1 oz)	42
Hummus-guacamole (2 tbsp)	50
Sweet Pea Guacamole (pg. 209; 1 tbsp)	21
Salsa (2 tbsp)	10
Hot sauce (1 tbsp)	1
Barbecue sauce (2 tbsp)	10
Ketchup (1 tbsp)	15
Mustard (1 tsp)	0
Vegan Mayo (pg. 262; 1 tbsp)	10
Vegan mayo (Nayonaise; 1 tbsp)	32
Vegan mayo (Vegenaise; 1 tbsp)	90
Corn (2 tbsp)	16
Hummus (2 tbsp)	45
Relish (1 tbsp)	5
Pickle Spear (1)	5

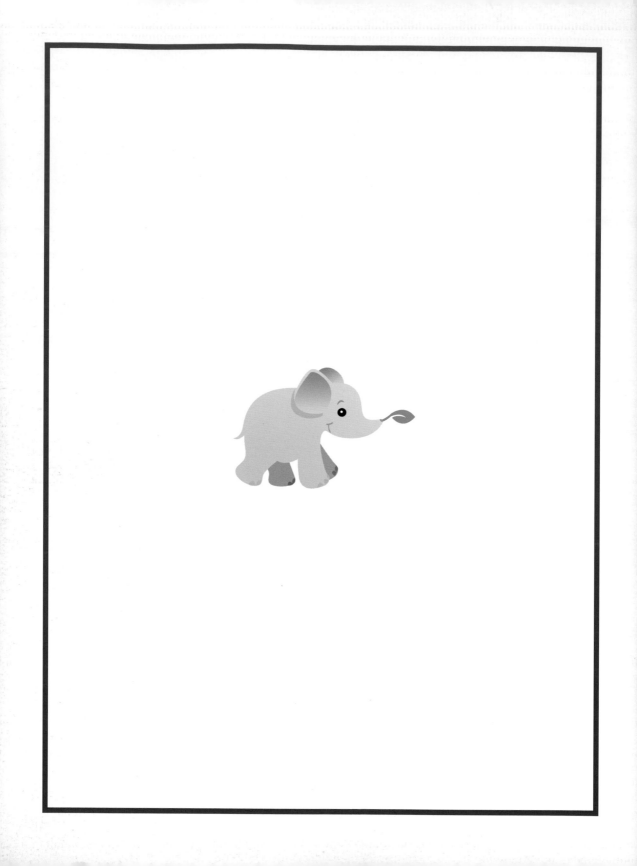

bowls & wraps

"Bowls" are one of the most popular food genres on my 7-Day Meal Plans because they're easy, fast, and fun. So what is a bowl?

It's typically a mix of greens, grains, legumes, and other vegetables or fruits in a bowl that can be served warm, room temp, or cold. My friend Kait describes them as "come-home-and-wash-something-and-then-open-a-bunch-of-stuff-from-my-pantry" dinners.

Wraps are also crazy popular on the **7-DAY MEAL PLANS** and for good reasons: They come together quickly, they're portable, and they have all the goodness of a salad but they feel like so much more than a salad! (AND they're often single-serving!) In this section, you'll find my favorite low calorie but satisfying

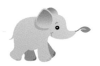

wraps inspired by the 7-Day Meal Plans—most are around 200 calories or less. Wraps make for a hearty snack, but they can become a meal if paired with soup, chili, salad, or fruit. Just roll them up and enjoy!

BONUS: Most of the "bowls" can also be turned into wraps and vice versa, giving you so many possibilities! You can also substitute the wrap with two slices of bread to make a sandwich or with two corn tortillas, but the nutritional value will vary slightly.

GLUTEN-FREE FOLKS: A brown rice tortilla (or two corn tortillas) is a fine substitution for a whole-wheat wrap, but you can also substitute ½ cup cooked quinoa to make a bowl or salad instead. (About 3 tbsp uncooked quinoa has the same caloric value as a wrap.)

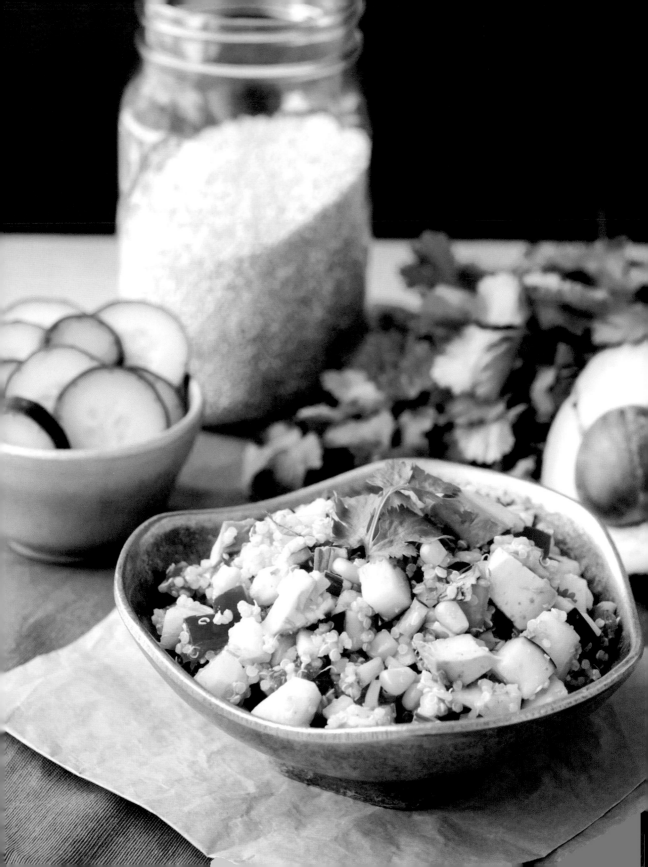

"cheater" ancient bowl

I've always been fascinated with ancient civilizations, particularly the Mayans, Incas, and Aztecs. Most of the ingredients in this bowl are borrowed from those early diets. I call this a "cheater" recipe since I use a bit of avocado, but you can omit the avocado (and perhaps replace it with sweet potato) if you want. I find the avocado lends a nice creamy element to the dish.

Toss all ingredients together, adding lime juice to taste as desired. (I also like to add hot sauce in addition to the lime sometimes.)

Chef's Note Jicama (sounds like *hick*-uh-muh) is a root vegetable and can be found at most supermarkets and all health food stores. It's one of my favorite snacks. After peeling it and chopping slices, try drizzling lime juice on it and add a dash of chili pepper or cayenne, if you dare!

PER BOWL

Calories	304
Fat	8.7g
Carbs	54.1g
Fiber	11.3g
Sugars	9.4g
Protein	9.5g
WW Points	8

SINGLE SERVING

½ c cooked quinoa

1 tomato, diced

½ cucumber, diced or sliced

½ c diced jicama

¼ c diced avocado

¼ c diced red onion

juice of 1 lime

⅓ c corn

1 tsp ground cumin

cilantro (optional)

UNDER 350 CALORIES

PER BOWL

Calories 330
Fat. 7.8g
Carbs 55.3g
Fiber 5.3g
Sugars. 7.7g
Protein 13.4g
WW Points 9

SINGLE SERVING

¼ c uncooked brown rice (or ¾ c already cooked)

½ c low-sodium vegetable broth

5 baby carrots, sliced into thin sticks

½ cucumber, diced

1 green onion, sliced

3 oz firm or extra-firm tofu, cubed

2 tbsp Thai Peanut Dressing (pg. 140)

1–2 tbsp crushed peanuts (optional)

cilantro (optional)

asian rice bowl

When my husband Scott and I were living in a small ski town in Colorado, our favorite place to eat out was at a fusion sushi place called Spostas. Unlike more traditional Japanese restaurants, this place did things like "cheeseburger" sushi. We loved going there because they offered a long list of ingredients, most of which were fruits and vegetables that could be used in any combination to design your own sushi or rice bowl. My sister's favorite combination was green apple and honey sushi (it's actually pretty good!) and I developed a love affair with cucumber and yellow bell pepper teriyaki sushi. Anyway, Scott doesn't "do" seaweed, so he always ordered a rice bowl. At home we re-created the rice bowl, only with a touch of Thai rather than Japanese. The dish is deliciously filling and so easy to make. Even if you have to make the sauce from scratch, you're still done as fast as you can whisk!

Combine rice with ½ cup vegetable broth, bring to a boil, cover and simmer until liquid has evaporated and rice is fluffy, or use about ¾ cup already cooked rice. Combine warm (or chilled) rice and carrots and remaining ingredients, drizzling Thai Peanut Dressing over top and garnishing with a few reserved green onion slices, plus peanuts and cilantro if using. (I also sometimes add Sriracha, an Asian hot sauce, and sweet red chili sauce over top.)

VARIATION

Make it a Wrap: Skip the rice and put all of the ingredients in a wrap with some shredded lettuce for 124 calories.

burrito bowl

This is one of my favorite "easy" meals when I'm exhausted after a long day but still want something with great flavor and texture. This bowl comes together in a snap and satisfies the hungriest of bellies. For an even more filling meal, try adding in some leftover brown rice.

Place cold lettuce in a bowl. Top with warmed vegetarian refried beans, diced chilled tomato, green onion, corn, and black olives. Add salsa on top (as a dressing), plus hot sauce as desired (I use 2–3 tbsp) and avocado or guacamole, if using.

VARIATION

Make it a Wrap: Divide ingredients between two wraps for approximately 293 calories each.

PER BOWL

Calories	337
Fat	6.4g
Carbs	60g
Fiber	18.5g
Sugars	12.7g
Protein	17.3g
WW Points	8

SINGLE SERVING

- 4 c chopped lettuce
- ¾ c vegetarian refried beans
- 1 tomato, diced
- 2 green onions, sliced
- ⅓ c corn
- 3 tbsp sliced black olives
- ½ c salsa
  hot sauce, as desired
  avocado or guacamole (optional)

caribbean bowl

PER BOWL

Calories	347
Fat	3.9g
Carbs	65.6g
Fiber	12.6g
Sugars	8.3g
Protein	16.7g
WW Points	9

I love the pairing of black beans and pineapple! Inspired by the Caribbean Chili (pg. 116), now you have a Caribbean Bowl too! Avocado and guacamole also make a nice addition.

SINGLE SERVING

- 2 c kale, chopped
- ½ c cooked quinoa
- ½ c black beans
- ½ c pineapple salsa
- ½ c diced or crushed pineapple
- 2 green onions, sliced

Line a pot with a thin layer of water, bring to a boil, add kale, and cover for about a minute (the kale will turn bright green). Give it a stir so all of the kale is bright green and softer, then drain. Mix in quinoa and/or beans to warm it up a bit, if desired. (I like to serve this with everything warm except the salsa, pineapple, and green onion, which are chilled.) Transfer to a bowl and toss with salsa, pineapple, and green onions, leaving a few onion pieces for garnish. You can also drizzle hot sauce on top if desired.

VARIATION

Make it a Wrap: Divide ingredients (skipping quinoa and using spinach instead of kale) into two wraps, for approximately 196 calories each.

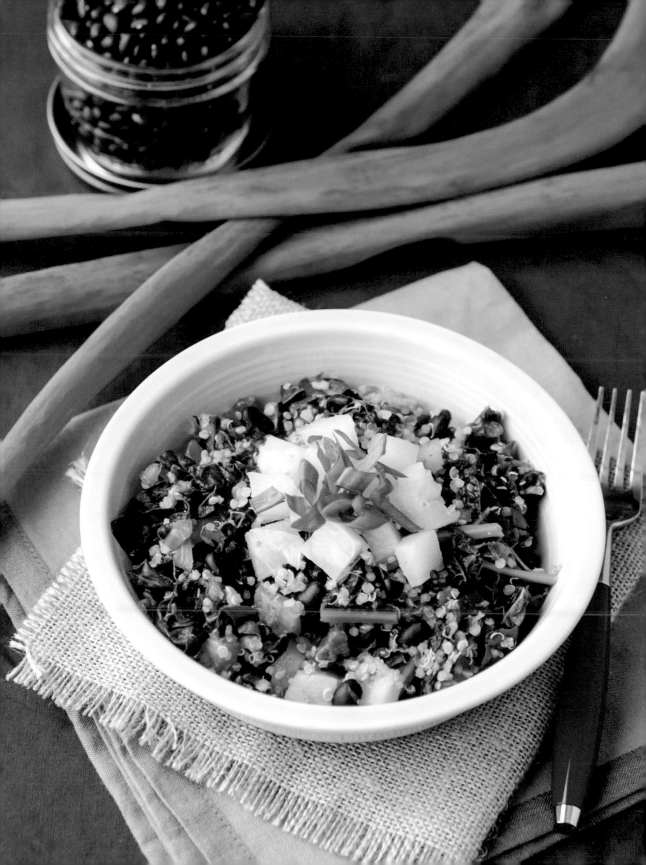

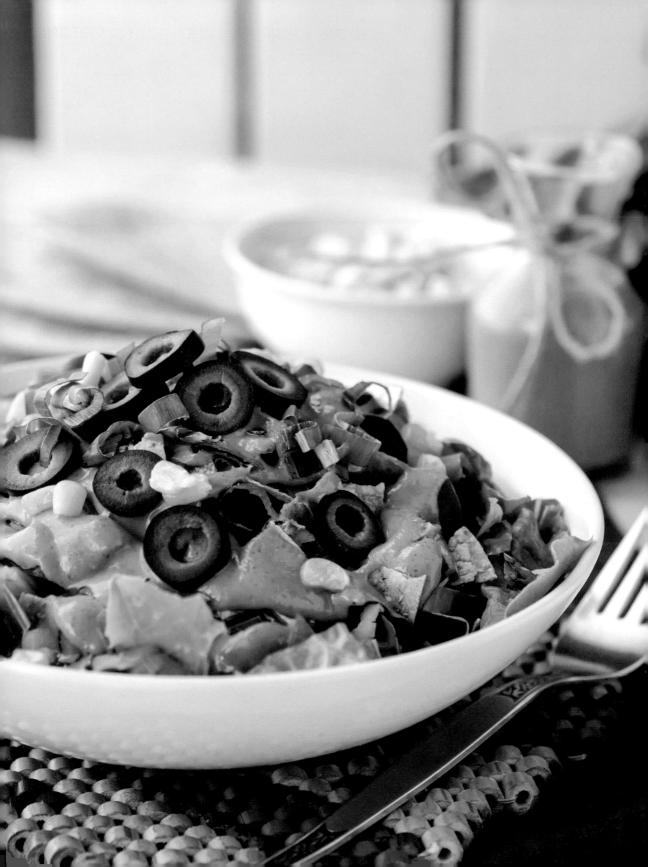

nacho bowl

We love nachos and I tend to make them any night we want a fast, easy, and quick meal. Which means I make nachos pretty often. Problem is, even with homemade baked corn chips (corn tortillas cut and crisped in the oven), the caloric value is pretty high. That's when I started considering "nacho" salads as an alternative with a better caloric density. It has all the taste of nachos with the healthy goodness of a salad—*and* is mindful of calories. Win-win! Fill up, feel great, and scratch the nacho itch!

Crisp corn tortilla in an oven or toaster oven for a few minutes at 350°F. Meanwhile, prepare or re-warm nacho sauce. Add cool lettuce to a bowl, top with black beans, corn (I love using roasted corn from Trader Joe's here), tomato, and green onion slices (saving a few for garnish). Crumble crisped tortilla over salad and smother with nacho sauce. Garnish with reserved green onion and black olive slices, if desired.

PER BOWL

Calories	301
Fat	4.3g
Carbs	54.8g
Fiber	15.9g
Sugars	9.7g
Protein	18g
WW Points	7

SINGLE SERVING

- 1 corn tortilla
- 1 serving Quick Nacho Sauce (pg. 212)
- 4 c chopped or shredded lettuce
- ¼ c black beans
- ¼ c corn
- ½ tomato, diced
- 1 green onion, sliced
  black olives, sliced (optional)
  hot sauce (optional)
  lime juice (optional)

Chef's Note I sometimes toss my beans with a little hot sauce and my tomatoes with a little lime juice for added flavor intensity. By the way, pinto beans work great, too.

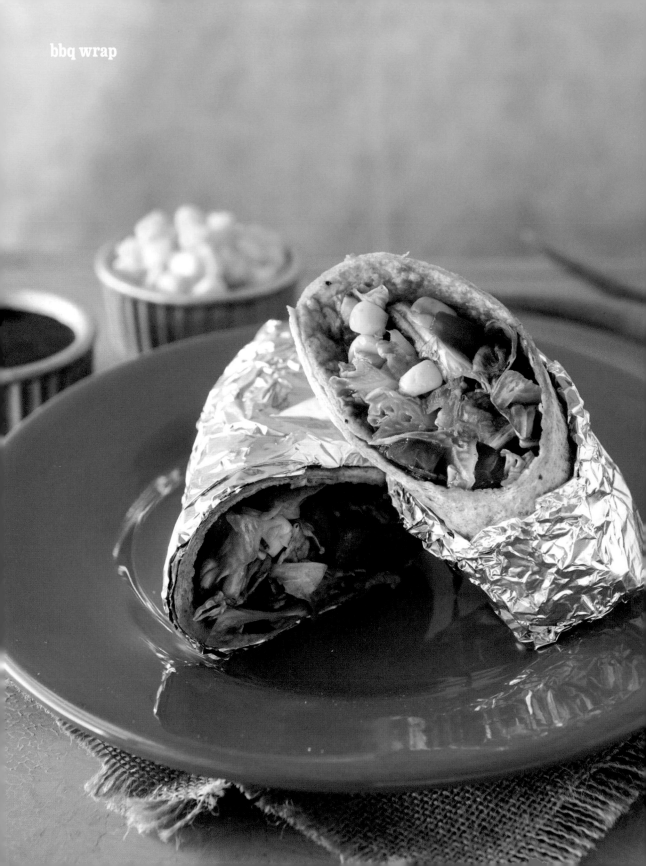

bbq wrap

italian bowl

If you've never had broccoli with marinara before—prepare to have your world rocked! Seriously! So simple and yet so-crazy-delicious. To extend this dish, slip in some white beans such as cannellini. You can add ¼ cup white beans for just 50 extra calories.

Cook pasta al dente (firm but not too hard), and rinse. Combine cooked pasta with steamed/cooked broccoli and warmed marinara. Sprinkle generously with Parmesan and serve.

Chef's Note To make this gluten-free, use brown rice pasta or another gluten-free pasta in place of the whole-wheat.

PER SERVING
ITALIAN BOWL / BBQ WRAP

Calories 294/200
Fat 2.5g/1.7g
Carbs 57.3g/43.8g
Fiber 9.1g/5.1g
Sugars 13.4g/16g
Protein 17.9g/4.1g
WW Points 6/5

SINGLE SERVING

2 oz pasta (any kind; see note)

2 c broccoli florets, cooked

1 c marinara sauce, warmed

AJ's Vegan Parmesan (pg. 271)

bbq wrap

I could eat this wrap every day and never tire of it. Lettuce, barbecue sauce, and corn is my favorite combination—you might have noticed my BBQ Salad (pg. 133) too! For a bit of a crunch, add broken baked corn chips.

Toss vegetables with barbecue sauce until well coated. Place into wrap and roll up.

SINGLE SERVING

2 c lettuce, chopped

½ tomato, sliced

¼ c corn

1 green onion, sliced

3 tbsp barbecue sauce

1 wrap

PER WRAP
CLASSIC VEGGIE / ROASTED RED BELL PEPPER

Calories	207/278
Fat	5.6g/2g
Carbs	35.1g/56.2g
Fiber	7.3g/13.6g
Sugars	4.3g/11.7g
Protein	7.2g/11g
WW Points	5/7

SINGLE SERVING

1 wrap
3 tbsp hummus
  red onion, sliced
¼ cucumber, sliced
½ carrot, shredded
½ tomato, sliced

SINGLE SERVING

⅓ c cooked white beans
1 wrap
1 red onion, sliced
1 c spinach
½ carrot, shredded
1 roasted red pepper
  (in water, not oil),
  sliced

Chef's Note Any white beans—navy, cannellini, butter bean—will work in this recipe. You can also substitute red pepper hummus (3 tbsp) for the beans.

classic veggie wrap

Why spend five dollars or more on the go when you can make a fresh wrap at home for a fraction of the cost? Here's my basic veggie wrap, built on my overly simplified (but delightful) hummus wrap snack that's just a small tortilla, hummus, and spring mix greens, plus a little tomato if I have it on hand. You can also slip in spinach and use different hummus flavors, like red pepper hummus.

Slather hummus on wrap. Add onion, cucumber, shredded carrot, and tomato slices, plus a sprinkling of fresh black pepper if desired. Roll up and enjoy!

roasted red bell pepper wrap

I love roasted red bell peppers and this wrap lets them shine. The carrot adds a nice sweetness to the wrap and the white beans provide a little bulk and protein.

Mash beans with a fork and mix with salt and pepper to taste. Spread bean mixture on the wrap and then add red onion, spinach, shredded carrot, and roasted red pepper. Roll up and enjoy!

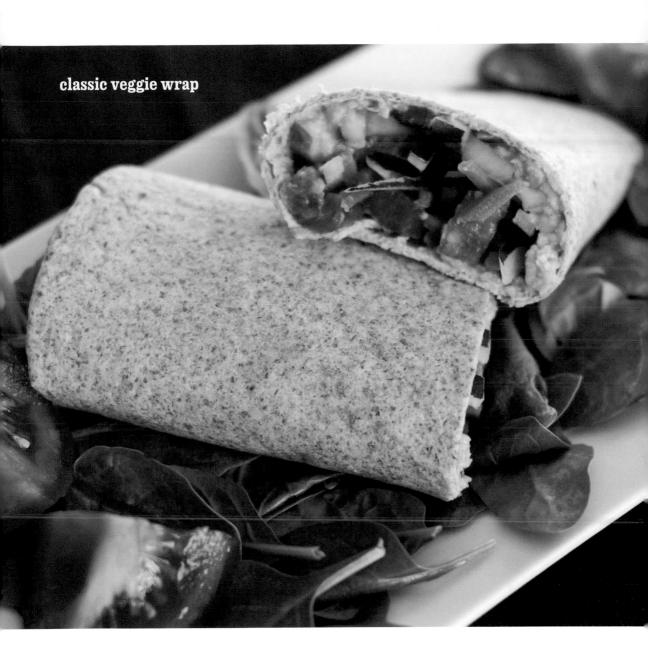

classic veggie wrap

UNDER 200 CALORIES

PER WRAP	
Calories	159
Fat	2g
Carbs	32.9g
Fiber	6.7g
Sugars	7.4g
Protein	4.9g
WW Points	4

MAKES 2

- 2 c spinach
- 1 tomato, sliced
- 1 roasted red bell pepper (in water, not oil), sliced
- 8 strawberries, sliced
- 2 wraps

Chef's Note For a twist, sometimes I leave off the bell pepper, add in some white beans, and drizzle a little balsamic vinegar or fat-free balsamic vinaigrette over the vegetables.

spinach love wrap

This is another wrap inspired by the 7-Day Meal Plans. I call this a spinach "love" wrap because of the strawberry "hearts." Plus it's so easy to make, it's only 159 calories per wrap, and its really filling. What's not to love?

Place spinach, tomato slices, bell pepper slices, and strawberry slices in each wrap and roll up.

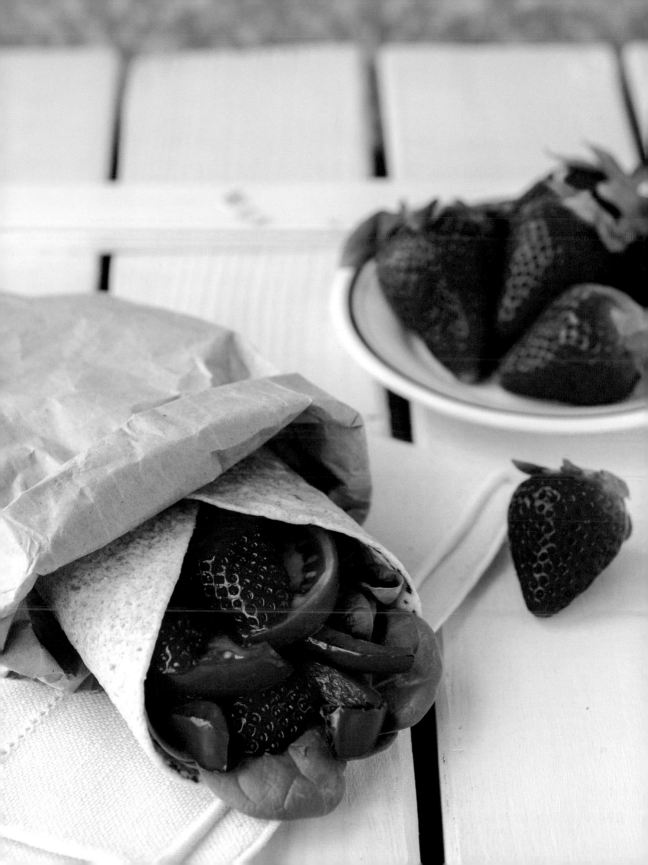

smashed white bean wrap

PER WRAP

Calories	350
Fat	8.8g
Carbs	58.9g
Fiber	17.3g
Sugars	1.2g
Protein	14.6g
WW Points	9

SINGLE SERVING

- ¾ c cooked white beans
- 2 oz guacamole or ¼ avocado
- 1 wrap
- red onion, sliced
- ¼ c spinach
- hot sauce (optional)
- sprouts (optional)

Chef's Notes

» Any white bean will work in this recipe—cannellini, navy, butter bean, etc.

» Wholly Guacamole sells guacamole in pre-portioned sizes of 2 oz, and you can freeze whatever you're not using!

The Smashed White Bean & Avocado Club is, hands down, the most beloved sandwich on the 7-Day Meal Plans. I knew I had to include it in this cookbook, so I modified it slightly and turned it into a wrap! It's a "cheater" recipe since I use a little avocado, but my, my, how far that little avocado goes in terms of taste!

Mash beans with a fork and mix with salt and pepper to taste. Mix in guacamole (or reserve for layering). Spread bean mixture on the wrap and then add red onion, spinach (add more than ¼ cup if you like), and guacamole if you haven't already used it. Drizzle with hot sauce if desired and top with sprouts if using. Roll up and enjoy!

scott's burrito

No one really needs a recipe for a burrito—but I wanted to share Scott's favorite (filling!) 200-calorie burrito. You see, I think my husband ate bean burritos for lunch every weekday for a year. Back when we were living in Manhattan, we struggled to make ends meet and packing a lunch was an easy way to save money. The problem Scott had was that his office had no fridge or microwave, and bean burritos were about the only food he didn't mind eating at room temperature. Even things like homemade burgers weren't an easy option because there were no condiments at work, and who wants a soggy bun? Anyway, Scott made subtle changes to his burrito day to day, but this combination was most popular, and remains a staple in his lunches today. The combination of whole-grain tortillas, beans, and vegetables helps keep him full. He packs three of these, plus fruit and another snack.

Combine vegetarian refried beans with salsa. Spread on tortilla. Top with corn, onion, spinach, and guacamole. Drizzle generously with hot sauce, roll up, and enjoy!

PER BURRITO

Calories	200
Fat	2.4g
Carbs	37.8g
Fiber	10g
Sugars	5.2g
Protein	10.3
WW Points	5

SINGLE SERVING

- ⅓ c vegetarian refried beans
- ¼ c salsa
- 1 whole-grain tortilla
- 2–3 tbsp corn
- 1 green onion or other onion, sliced
- 1 c spinach or lettuce
- 3 tbsp Sweet Pea Guacamole (pg. 209)
- hot sauce

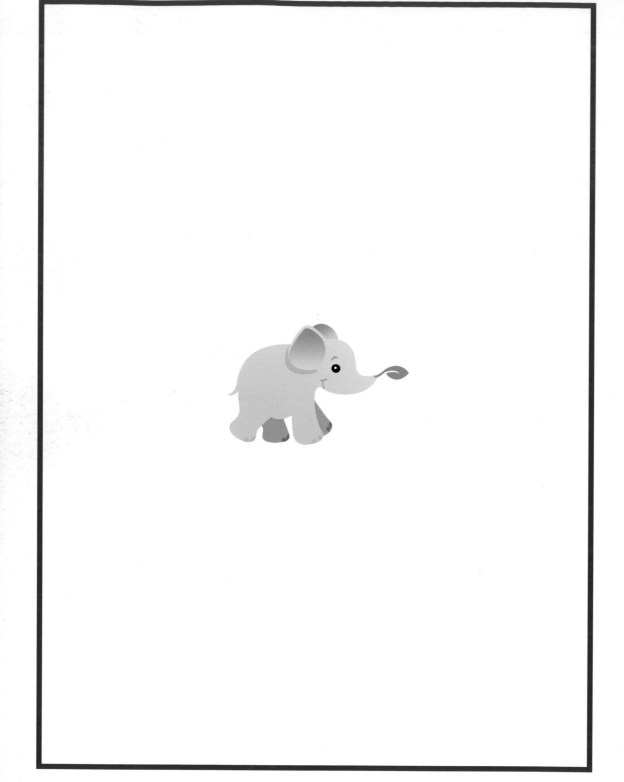

soups, stews & savory pies

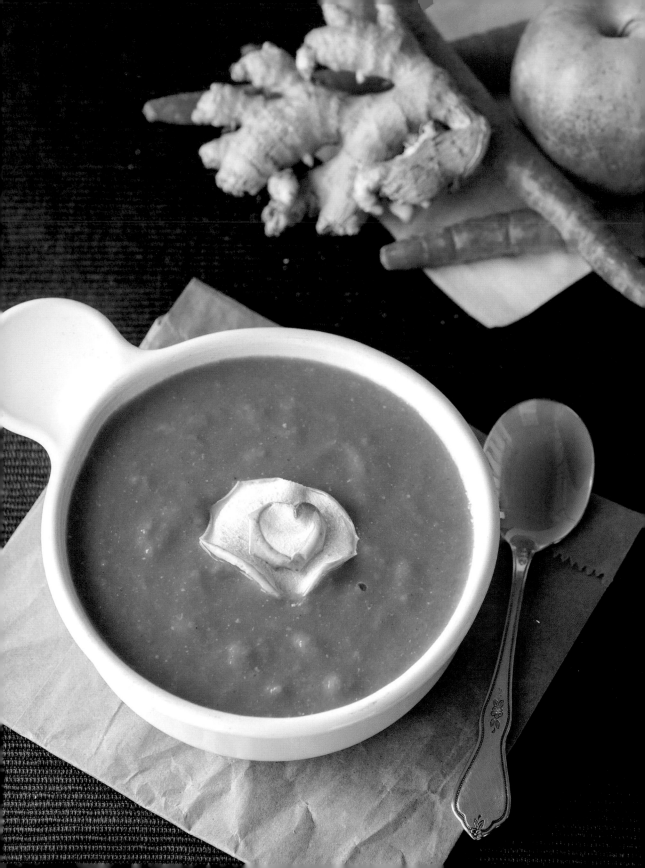

carrot soup

You can make this carrot soup two ways! It's an easy, light, and filling lunch when paired with a salad.

Line a saucepan with a thin layer of broth and sauté carrots over high heat until they start to soften, about 4 minutes. Add apples, plus more broth if needed, then reduce heat to medium and cover. Cook for another minute or two, until apples and carrots are fork-tender (apples will take on a golden yellow coloring). Transfer to a blender and blend until smooth, adding more broth as necessary—I usually add at least 1 cup. Return to pot. Stir in ¼ cup nondairy milk. Add curry powder or ground ginger to taste, starting with ¼ tsp. If you go overboard with the spice or your apple is too sweet, add more nondairy milk. Serve warm.

PER SERVING

Calories 236
Fat. 1.7g
Carbs 57.4g
Fiber 11.5g
Sugars. 32.5g
Protein 3g
WW Points 6

SINGLE SERVING

- 2 c vegetable broth
- 4 carrots, peeled and diced
- 1 red apple, cored and diced
- ¼ c nondairy milk
- mild yellow curry powder or ground ginger

I think what I love most about soups is how well they play into the goal of caloric density. First you have the broth, which is water-rich, and then you have the vegetables in the soup that are also water-rich and high in fiber. The result is a filling soup for fewer calories (that's also nutritious). More volume. More bulk. Fewer calories. A soup for the win!

butternut soup

PER SERVING

Calories 140
Fat 0.6g
Carbs 35.9g
Fiber 6.3g
Sugars 6.7g
Protein 3g
WW Points 4

SERVES 2

1 **butternut squash**

1 **c low-sodium vegetable broth**

2 **tsp mild yellow curry powder**

Divine simplicity. This soup has just three ingredients, but it's so delicious and surprisingly filling. Although this soup is a frequent fall and winter lunch for us (paired with a salad), I also like to serve it as a starter at Thanksgiving.

Preheat oven to 375°F. Slice butternut squash in half and place on a cookie sheet cut-side-down. Bake for 25–45 minutes, until you can easily stab it with a fork, but check regularly so you don't burn your squash. Remove from oven and let cool until it's safe to handle. Use a spoon to scoop out and remove seeds and strings, and discard them. Then spoon out butternut flesh into a blender. Combine with broth and curry powder. Whiz until smooth and silky, adding water or additional broth if necessary. Transfer to a saucepan and warm over low heat. Season with salt, if desired, and more curry to taste, if desired.

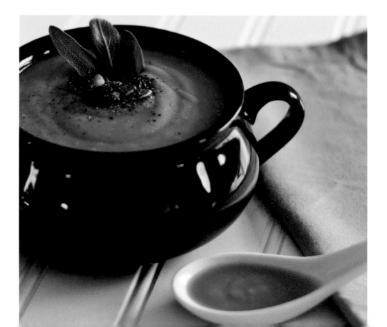

✓ SOY-FREE ✓ FAT-FREE ✓ QUICK ✓ BUDGET

carol's cabbage soup

This is my Aunt Carol's cabbage soup recipe made vegan—don't be alarmed by the big serving size! Although this recipe makes a lot of soup, there are so few calories per serving that you can have as many bowls as you like. (Just don't go all "cabbage soup diet" on me!) To bulk up this soup, I like to toss in leftover cooked grains such as brown rice or quinoa. Freeze leftovers!

Cut cabbage in half, then cut out the hard core at the bottom (discard or save for making vegetable broth). Chop remaining cabbage and set aside. Line a large pot with a thin layer of water or vegetable broth and sauté cabbage, celery, and onion until tender. Add water, bouillon, plus salt and pepper (Aunt Carol uses 1½ tsp each of salt and pepper), tomato sauce, sugar, and ketchup. Cover, bring to a boil, and then reduce heat to low and simmer for 10 minutes or until thoroughly heated.

PER SERVING
(ABOUT 1 CUP)

Calories 42
Fat 0.4g
Carbs 8.6g
Fiber 2.5g
Sugars 6g
Protein 2.2g
WW Points 1

SERVES 16

- 1 medium head cabbage
- 1 c chopped celery
- 1 c chopped onion
- 8 c water
- 1 no-beef bouillon cube (see Chef's Note)
- 2 15-oz cans tomato sauce
- 1 tbsp brown sugar
- ¼ c ketchup

Chef's Note You can skip the bouillon and replace 2 cups of water with 2 cups of No-Beef Broth (pg. 264). You can also find commercially made vegan "beef" bouillon cubes at well-stocked supermarkets and health food stores. Popular brands are Edward & Sons and Superior Touch's Better Than Bouillon.

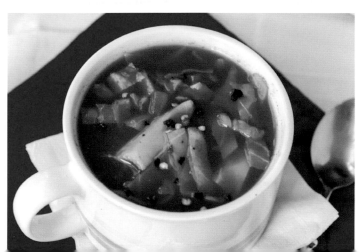

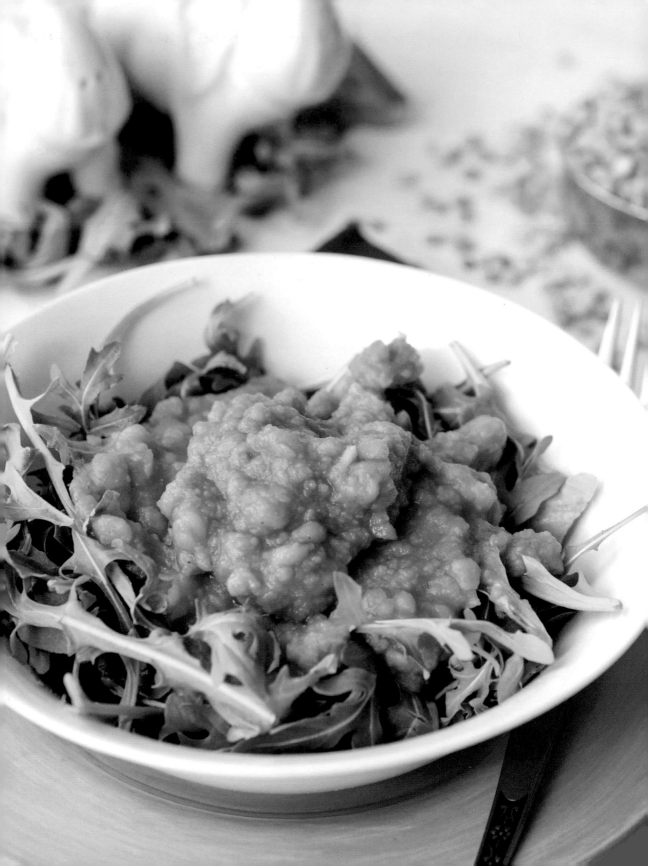

yellow curry dal

Simple and yet deliciously filling. I make this soup anytime I'm in need of a fast meal and both my pantry and fridge are looking pretty bare. This dal is also great over greens (treat it like a gravy!).

Combine split peas with 1 cup broth and cover. Bring to a boil then immediately reduce heat to low and simmer until water has evaporated. Add another ½ cup broth, cover again, and bring to a boil, then reduce heat to low and simmer until water has evaporated. Use a potato masher to mash up some of the split peas and make it creamier (you can also use an immersion blender briefly, or transfer part to a blender). Then add the last ¼ cup broth, plus ½ tsp curry powder. Stir to combine. Taste, adding more curry powder if desired (some curries are hotter than others). Add salt to taste, if desired, and serve.

PER SERVING

Calories 177
Fat 0.6g
Carbs 32g
Fiber 12.7g
Sugars 4.4g
Protein 12.2g
WW Points 4

SERVES 2

½ c uncooked yellow split peas

1¾ c vegetable broth, divided

½ –1 tsp mild yellow curry powder

celeriac soup

Celeriac is the fancier term for celery root—the ugliest root at the market (it looks like a space creature, in my opinion). But pureed into a soup? Oh-so-creamy and delicious.

PER SERVING

Calories 305
Fat. 2.9g
Carbs 69.1g
Fiber. 12.4g
Sugars. 29.6g
Protein 6.9g
WW Points. 8

SINGLE SERVING

- 1 c vegetable broth
- 1 onion, diced
- 1 celery root, peeled and diced
- 1–2 green apples, cored and diced
- ½ –1 c nondairy milk
- 1 tbsp pure maple syrup (optional)
- smoked paprika
- Tempeh Bacon (pg. 36) (optional)

Chef's Note Almond or soy milk work best in this recipe since they are so creamy.

Line a medium pot with a thin layer of broth and sauté onion over high heat for a minute. Add celery root and more broth if necessary, and sauté until the celery root starts to soften, about 3 minutes. Add 1 green apple (diced) and more broth if necessary, and reduce heat to medium. Sauté for another minute or two, until celery root is fork-tender and brown in color and the apples have softened. Transfer to a food processor or blender and add ½ cup nondairy milk. Blend until smooth and creamy, adding more nondairy milk as necessary to achieve a soup consistency. Allow the soup to cool (so it's warm but not lava hot) and taste. If you'd like a stronger apple flavor, transfer ¾ of the soup back to the pot, adding the second apple (diced) with the remaining soup in the blender, and blend. Then mix in with soup in your pot. Taste, adding maple syrup to taste if desired, plus salt and pepper. Heat over low if you need to warm it up again. Garnish with smoked paprika and chopped tempeh bacon, if using. I also like to leave a celery leaf on top to make it look fancy.

cajun corn chowder

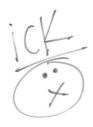

One of my go-to quick lunches is a creamy corn soup that uses frozen corn blended in part with nondairy milk and a touch of chipotle powder—that's it! One day I grabbed Cajun seasoning by mistake and had myself a delicious accident.

Warm corn or let it thaw. Transfer 1 cup corn to a blender with nondairy milk and cornstarch, and blend until smooth or pulpy (your choice!). Transfer to a saucepan and stir in remaining corn, 1 tbsp ketchup, and several dashes of seasoning. Bring to a boil then reduce heat to low, stirring until it's thick and chowder-like. Taste, adding more ketchup (I like just a hint of tomato, but a strong tomato flavor is good, too—my testers all seemed to prefer 2 tbsp) and more seasoning to taste (I use about 1 tsp).

Stews, chilis, etc. are great because they load you up with vegetables and beans that are both high in fiber and water-rich, making them very filling and satisfying, too.

PER SERVING

Calories	350
Fat	6.7g
Carbs	71.6g
Fiber	9.4g
Sugars	13.3g
Protein	11.2g
WW Points	10

SINGLE SERVING

- 2 c frozen corn, divided
- 1 c nondairy milk
- 1 tbsp cornstarch
- 1–3 tbsp ketchup
- Cajun seasoning (see Chef's Note) or Old Bay Seasoning

Chef's Note To make Cajun seasoning yourself, blend 2 tbsp sweet paprika, 2 tbsp granulated garlic powder, 1 tbsp cayenne pepper, 1 tbsp chili powder, 1 tbsp pepper, 1 tbsp dried oregano or marjoram, 1 tbsp granulated onion powder, and ½ tsp ground nutmeg or mace (optional).

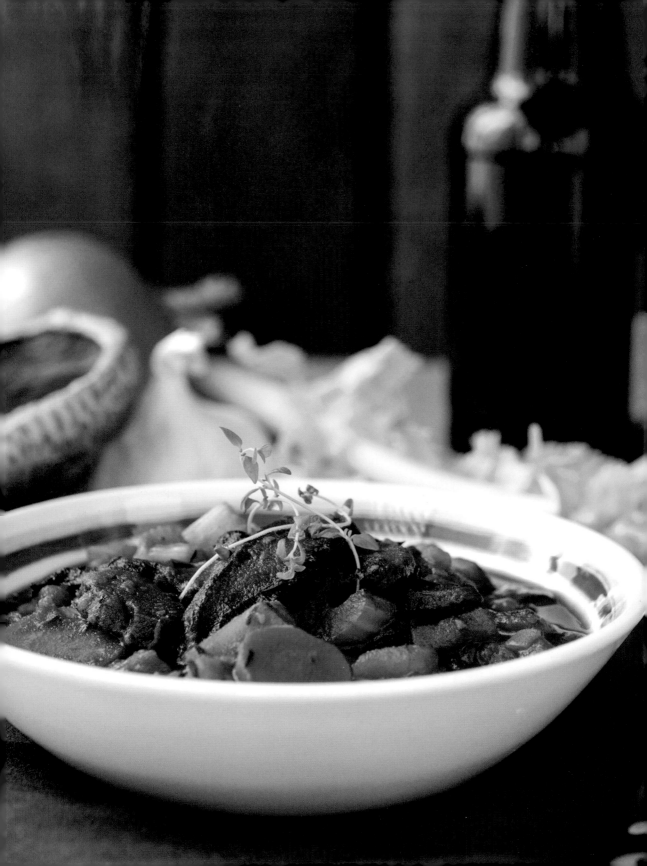

irish stew

When I was in Ireland, I saw signs all over for Irish stew and Guinness stew. My husband was intrigued and asked me to try a meat-free version when we got home. After scouring the Internet for traditional recipes, I came up with this healthy plant-based rendition. It's one of our favorite stews! It's got that "stick-to-your-ribs" satisfaction.

Remove stems from portobello mushrooms and discard. Cut mushroom caps into strips and set aside. Line a large pot with 1 cup no-beef broth. Sauté onion and garlic over high heat until onions are translucent, about a minute or two. Add thyme, carrots, celery, potatoes, stout, and tomato paste, and stir. Bring to a boil, cover, reduce heat to low, and continue to cook for about 10 minutes. Add mushrooms on top, along with Dijon, bay leaves, 1 tbsp Worcestershire sauce, and remaining broth. Bring to a boil again, cover and simmer for at least 30 minutes, stirring every so often. Continue to cook until mushrooms and potatoes are very soft—past fork-tender. Taste, adding more Worcestershire sauce if desired. Add a generous amount of black pepper and salt if desired. Remove bay leaves and serve.

PER SERVING
(1¾ CUPS)

Calories 112
Fat 0.9g
Carbs 19.7g
Fiber 3.8g
Sugars 3.6g
Protein 4.8g
WW Points 3

SERVES 3–4

- 2 portobello mushrooms
- 2 c No-Beef Broth (pg. 264), divided
- 1 onion, diced
- 4 garlic cloves, minced
- 4 thyme twigs, fresh, de-stemmed or 1–2 tsp dried thyme
- 2 large carrots, peeled and chopped
- 2 celery stalks, sliced
- 2 medium white potatoes, diced
- 1 c Guinness stout
- 2 tbsp tomato paste
- 1 tbsp Dijon mustard
- 2–3 bay leaves
- 1–2 tbsp Vegan Worcestershire Sauce (pg. 266)

Chef's Note You can substitute about 16 baby carrots for the 2 large carrots in this recipe.

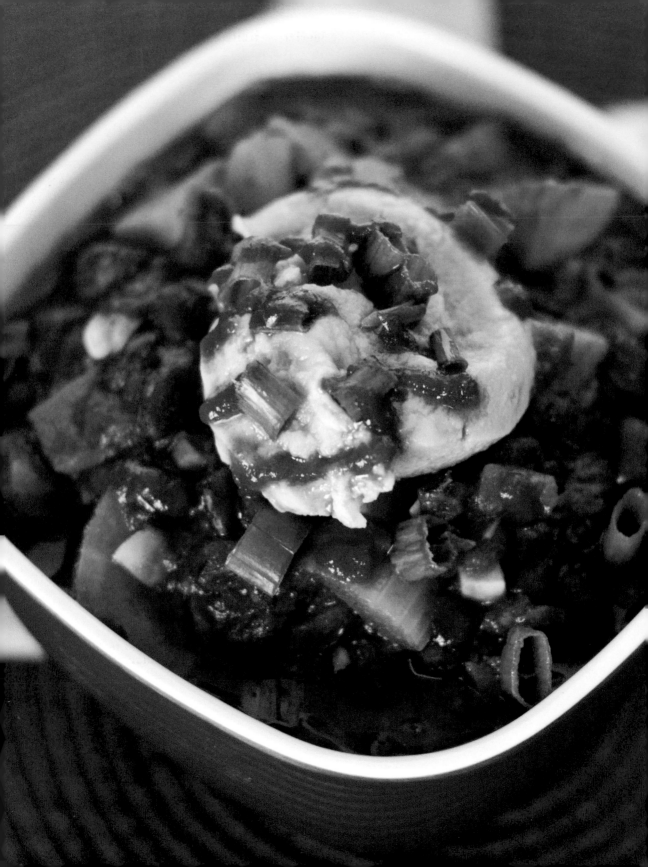

chipotle harvest chili

Sweet potatoes, kale, black beans, chipotle—this chili redefines chili! Serve with Classic Cornbread (pg. 55).

Line a large pot with a thin layer of broth, and sauté onion and garlic over high heat until translucent. Add remaining broth, sweet potato, tomato paste, a few light dashes of chipotle (a little goes a long way!), chili powder, and ground cumin. Cover, bring to a boil, and simmer until vegetables are fork-tender. Add corn, kale, and black beans with their liquid, stirring until the kale turns bright green, then darker green, and softens up. Add more chipotle to taste, if desired, and add more water or broth if you prefer your chili a bit soupier. Add ketchup and juice of ½ lime and stir. Serve with lime wedge for additional juicing at serving. Garnish with green onion and a dash of chipotle or smoked paprika.

PER SERVING
(1 CUP)

Calories 228
Fat. 2.2g
Carbs 45g
Fiber 10.1g
Sugars 9.4g
Protein 11.1g
WW Points 6

SERVES 2–3

1 c vegetable broth, divided
1 onion, diced
4 garlic cloves, minced
1 sweet potato, diced
6 tbsp tomato paste
chipotle powder
1 tbsp chili powder
1½ tsp ground cumin
1 c frozen corn
2 c chopped kale
1 15-oz can black beans, undrained
2 tbsp ketchup
1 lime
green onion
smoked paprika (optional)

Chef's Note No-salt-added/ unsalted beans are preferable here since you're not rinsing the beans.

Delicious!

PER SERVING

Calories	308
Fat	2.5g
Carbs	59.9g
Fiber	16.4g
Sugars	17.2g
Protein	16.3g
WW Points	7

SERVES 2

- ½ onion, diced
- 1 bell pepper (any), seeded and diced
- 1 c frozen pineapple chunks
- ½ c pineapple salsa
- 1 15-oz can black beans, drained and rinsed
- 1½ tsp chili powder
- 1 8-oz can tomato sauce
- hot sauce or cayenne, to taste
- brown sugar
- green onions, sliced (garnish)
- lime slices (optional)

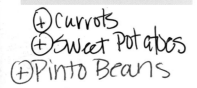
(+) carrots
(+) Sweet Potatoes
(+) Pinto Beans

caribbean chili

I don't actually remember eating chili the entire time I lived in the Caribbean, but I always seem to go with the name "Caribbean [Food]" when black beans and pineapple show up together. I love this tropical take on chili—warm pineapple adds an exciting twist. For a spicy kick, try adding a sliced or minced jalapeño.

Line a small saucepan with a thin layer of water or broth. Add onion and bell pepper, and sauté over high heat until bell pepper is bright and softer and onion is translucent, about 3 minutes. Add pineapple, salsa, beans, chili powder, and tomato sauce, and stir to combine. Cook for a minute or so until warm, then transfer ½ cup (or more) to a blender and process until smooth or partly smooth (adding a splash of water or broth if necessary). Stir blended chili into remaining chili and add hot sauce or cayenne to taste. You can also add a little brown sugar if you'd like a slight sweetness. (Sugar helps the pineapple flavor pop.) Add salt to taste then heat over low until thoroughly warm. Let chili rest 10 minutes so the flavors can merge. Serve topped with green onion and a lime garnish (squeezing lime juice over top, if desired).

Chef's Notes

» I always use frozen pineapple chunks in this recipe, but canned or fresh should also work.

» Red, white, sweet, Spanish—pretty much any kind of onion will work here. Use whatever you've got!

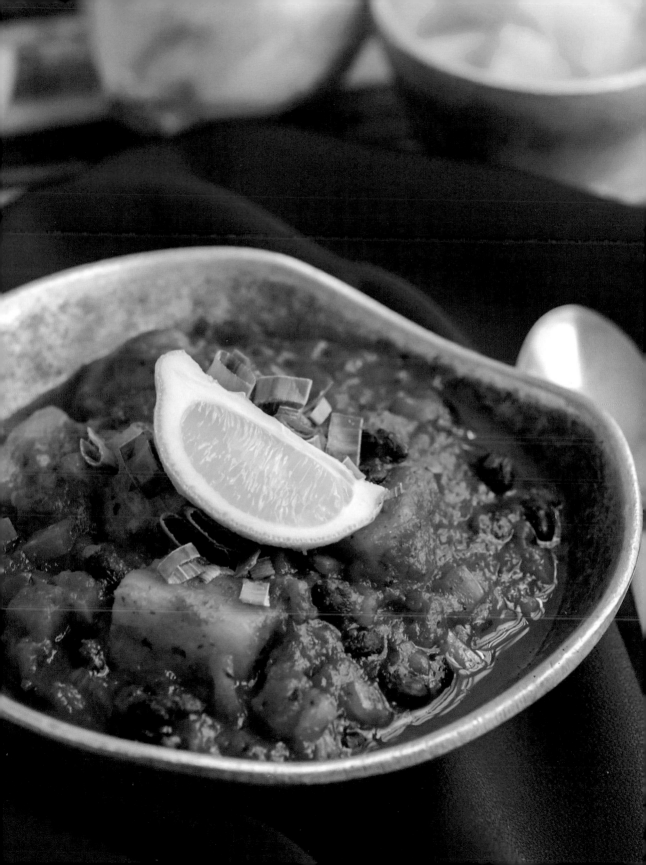

pumpkin chili

PER SERVING

Calories 262
Fat. 1.5g
Carbs 48.4g
Fiber 22.5g
Sugars. 6g
Protein 18g
WW Points. 5

SERVES 2

1 onion, diced

4 garlic cloves, minced

1 tbsp chili powder

1 tsp ground cumin

½ c low-sodium
   vegetable broth

½ c pure pumpkin
   (canned)

¼ c diced green chilies
   (canned)

2 tbsp tomato paste

1 15-oz can kidney or
   black beans, drained
   and rinsed

Chef's Note Black beans are
a fine substitution for the
kidney beans if that's all you
have on hand.

I love serving this chili in sugar pumpkins during the fall. There is something about serving food in another food that's just cool. This chili is also one of the most popular and beloved recipes in our fall 7-Day Meal Plans, so I just had to include it in this book.

Line a skillet with a thin layer of water, and sauté onion and garlic until onion is translucent, about 2–3 minutes. Add chili powder and ground cumin, stirring to coat onion, and continue to cook until all liquid has cooked off. Add broth, pumpkin, green chilies, and tomato paste, stirring to combine. Add beans and stir. Reduce heat to low and cook until beans are warm. Taste, adding salt and pepper, plus more spices, if desired. If it's too thick, thin out with water or vegetable broth.

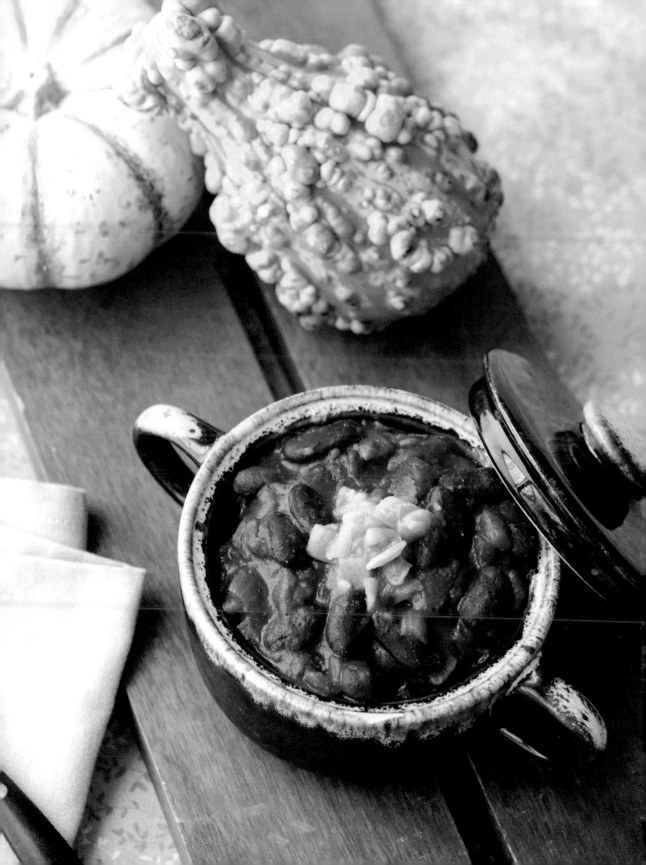

garden chili

I love this spicy chili because it celebrates vegetables, as opposed to most vegetarian chilis, which focus mainly on beans. This chili also looks quite stunning—perfect for dazzling guests on a cool or rainy night. Serve with Classic Cornbread (pg. 55) and be stuffed!

Line a large pot with a thin layer of broth, and sauté onion and garlic over high heat until onion is translucent, about a minute. Add bell pepper, tomatoes with juice, mushrooms, celery, carrots, tomato paste, remaining broth, spices, and condiments. Stir, cover, and bring to a boil. Once boiling, reduce to low and simmer until the vegetables are fork-tender, about 10 minutes. Add water or tomato sauce to make it more chili-like if necessary. Add beans and serve.

Chef's Note My friend Kim sent this recipe in her teenage daughter Brenna's lunch. Brenna's very-omni best friend said the following to Kim after school: "I LOVED that chili you tested for your friend. I just convinced myself to take a bite and get it over with so I wouldn't hurt Brenna's feelings. I have never tasted anything so good; when that book comes out next December, I am buying it myself and making that chili every single day for the rest of my life!" Teenager-tested and omni-approved!

PER SERVING
(1 CUP)

Calories 153
Fat. 1g
Carbs 30.5g
Fiber 12g
Sugars. 8.7g
Protein 9g
WW Points 3

SERVES 2–3

- 2 c vegetable broth, divided
- 1 onion, diced
- 4 garlic cloves, minced
- 1 green bell pepper, seeded and diced
- 1 15-oz can diced tomatoes (undrained)
- 1 c sliced mushrooms
- 2 celery stalks, sliced
- 2 carrots, peeled and diced
- ¼ c tomato paste
- 2 tbsp chili powder
- 1 tbsp Vegan Worcestershire Sauce (pg. 266)
- ½ tsp ground cumin
- 1 tbsp yellow mustard
- 1 15-oz can pinto or kidney beans, drained and rinsed

leftovers potpie

I call this "Leftovers" Potpie because it uses up your left-over vegetables and beans—a healthy and comforting way to clean out the fridge.

Preheat oven to 425°F and set aside a standard 9-inch bread pan. Line a skillet or large pot with ½ cup vegetable broth and sauté vegetables until fork-tender (and any frozen vegetable is thawed). Meanwhile, whisk nondairy milk, flour, nutritional yeast, and sage together. Pour over cooked veggies and bring to a near-boil. Reduce heat to low, stir, and simmer until thick and gravy-like. Add salt and pepper to taste. If it gets too thick, you can add a little more broth, but you want the veggies coated more than swimming. Pour vegetable mixture into bread pan and set aside. For biscuit topping, in a mixing bowl, whisk flour and baking powder together, then add milk and whisk again. Pour on top of vegetable mixture and use a spoon or spatula to spread the batter out evenly. Bake 10–15 minutes or until crust is golden and cooked through.

PER SERVING

Calories 314
Fat. 4.2g
Carbs 57.9g
Fiber 20.3g
Sugars. 1.4g
Protein 14.2g
WW Points 7

SERVES 2

½ –1 c vegetable broth

3 c leftover vegetables (chopped) and beans (see Chef's Note)

1 c nondairy milk

1½ tbsp white whole-wheat flour

1½ tbsp nutritional yeast

1 tsp rubbed sage (not powdered)

BISCUIT TOPPING

½ c white whole-wheat flour

½ tsp baking powder

½ c nondairy milk

Chef's Note I tend to use classic potpie vegetables like peas, corn, carrots, parsnips, and celery, plus beans like chickpeas or white beans. Even a frozen mix of vegetables would work.

PER SERVING
WITHOUT/WITH MASHED POTATOES

Calories	185/328
Fat	0.9g/2g
Carbs	33.8g/64g
Fiber	13.2g/17.6g
Sugars	7.5g/8.4g
Protein	12.1g/16.4
WW Points	4/8

SERVES 2

- 1 c No-Beef Broth (pg. 264), divided
- ½ small onion, diced
- 2 carrots, peeled and diced
- ½ c frozen peas
- ½ c cooked lentils
- 1 tsp cornstarch
- 2 tbsp tomato sauce
- 1–2 tsp Vegan Worcestershire Sauce (pg. 266)
- ⅛ tsp mild yellow curry powder
- Easy Mashed Potatoes (pg. 187)

shep's pie

This shepherd's pie is lentil-based, easy to make, filling, and, most importantly, fantastically delicious. It'll be in your regular rotation soon enough!

Line a skillet with a thin layer of broth. Add onion and carrots, and sauté over high heat until carrots become fork-tender, about 2–3 minutes. Add peas, and additional broth if necessary, and continue to cook until peas are warm, about a minute. Stir in lentils. Whisk cornstarch into remaining broth (about ½ cup) and pour into skillet. Stir in tomato sauce, plus 1 tsp Worcestershire sauce, and continue to cook, stirring, until it thickens. Taste, adding more Worcestershire sauce if desired, plus salt and pepper to taste. Stir in curry powder, then spoon into individual ramekins or small bowls and top with mashed potatoes. If crispy-topped mashed potatoes are desired, bake for a few minutes at 350°F, but this is not necessary.

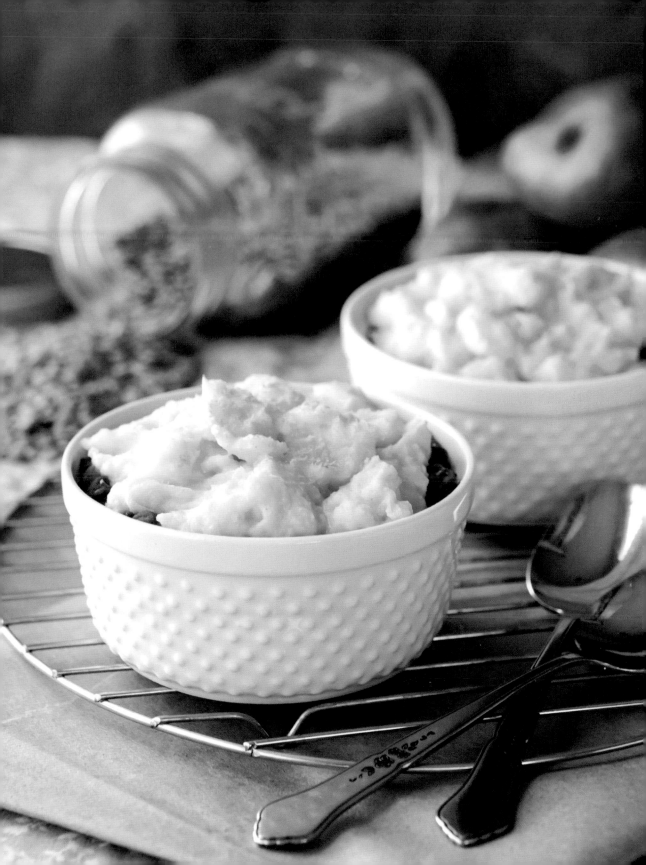

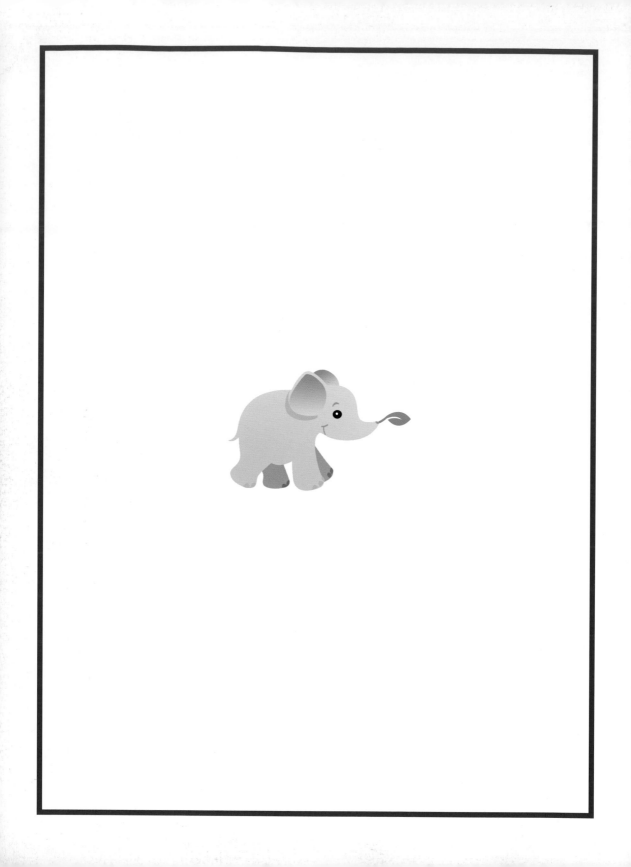

salads & dressings

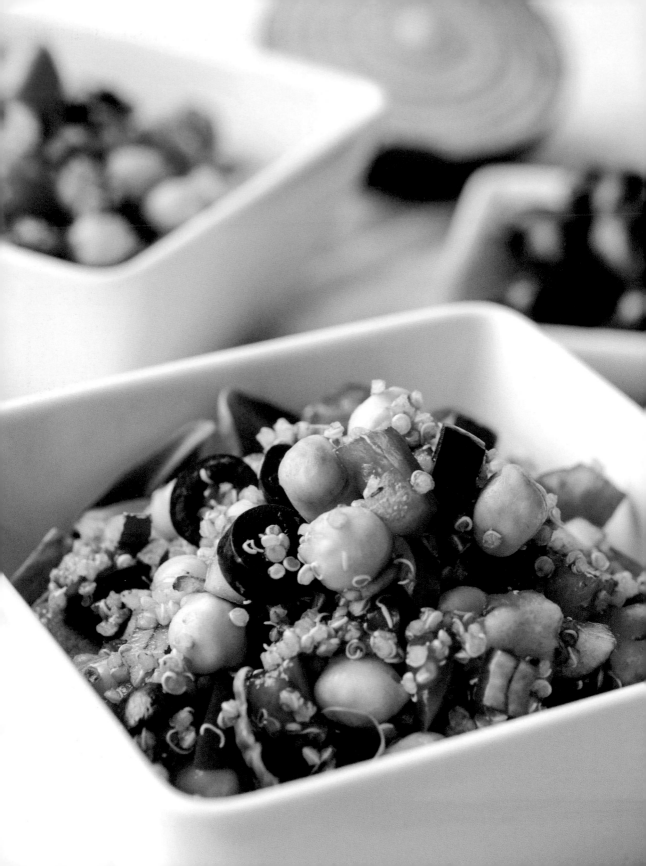

mediterranean quinoa salad

All my favorite Mediterranean flavors come together in this filling salad: olives, balsamic, fresh oregano—yum! Serve as a light side for two or enjoy as a meal for one.

In a medium saucepan, combine quinoa with broth, plus a splash of liquid from the olive jar. Cover, bring to a boil, then immediately reduce heat to low, and simmer until quinoa is fluffy and liquid has evaporated, about 15 minutes.

Once quinoa is cooked, toss it (warm or chilled) with ¼ cup sliced kalamata olives and the remaining ingredients, starting with 1 tbsp balsamic vinegar and adding more lemon zest, balsamic, or olive juice to taste.

I love a good salad and try to have one every day for my health. A daily salad helps ensure I'm eating greens and other vegetables regularly, and I also find I feel my best on days I've had a big ol' salad as a snack or side.

PER SERVING

Calories 177
Fat. 3.5g
Carbs 27g
Fiber 5.3g
Sugars. 1.3g
Protein 7.5g
WW Points. 4

SERVES 2

¼ c uncooked quinoa

½ c low-sodium vegetable broth

¼ c sliced kalamata olives, plus brine

1 tbsp balsamic vinegar

1 tomato, diced

lemon zest

fresh oregano (optional)

¼ c finely diced red onion

½ c chickpeas

2 c baby spinach

Chef's Note The quinoa can be served warm or cool. You can also serve the quinoa mixture over a bed of raw spinach, tossed with raw spinach, or if you prefer cooked spinach, stir it in with the hot quinoa as it finishes; it will cook, break down, and become softer. I prefer everything chilled.

lentil & pear salad

PER SERVING

Calories	340
Fat	0.9g
Carbs	65.1g
Fiber	25.7g
Sugars	15g
Protein	20.2g
WW Points	7

SINGLE SERVING

- 4 c salad mix (e.g., spring mix)
- 1 pear, sliced or diced
- 1 c cooked lentils
- Balsamic-Dijon Vinaigrette (pg. 137) or raspberry vinaigrette dressing
- ¼ red onion (optional), sliced thin

This recipe was born out of starvation. I was famished but the contents of my fridge were looking pretty bare: leftover salad mix, leftover lentils, a pear. . . . Hungry and with no other options, I put them all together, adding a little balsamic vinaigrette. I took one bite and went straight to heaven. I even patted myself on the back all the way to the kitchen for a second helping. This salad now appears regularly in my lunch rotation.

In a bowl, top salad mix with pear slices and lentils, then drizzle with dressing.

I tell users of my 7-Day Meal Plans to always order a full-size vegetable salad (with minimal dressing or just vinegar) as an appetizer when they have to (or want to) eat out. It helps fill you up before the rich restaurant main dish—keeping that balance.

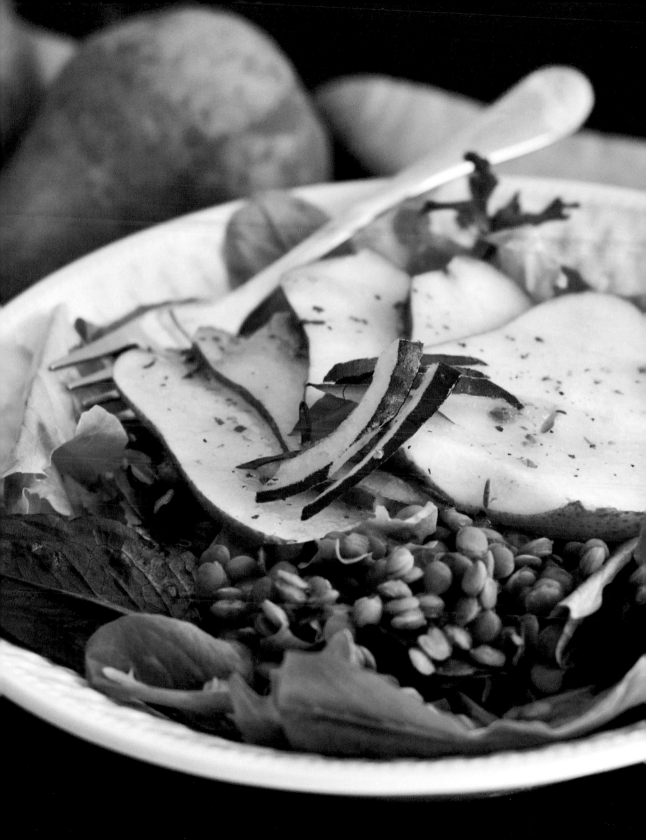

✔✔ SOY-FREE ✔✔ GLUTEN-FREE ✔✔ QUICK ✔ BUDGET ✔ SINGLE SERVING

UNDER
350
CALORIES

ONLY
300
CALORIES

waldorf salad

The Waldorf salad was created in the late 1800s at the Waldorf Hotel in New York City. Traditionally, it consists of apples, celery, and walnuts tossed with mayonnaise and served over a bed of crisp lettuce. Here's my lighter rendition that's easy to make and satisfying.

Toss apple, celery, chickpeas, and grapes together. Add 2 tbsp yogurt and toss to coat. Add another 1 tbsp of yogurt if necessary (everything should be lightly coated). Serve over lettuce.

tropical taco salad

Come summertime, this is one of the most requested salads on the 7-Day Meal Plans. I can't get enough of it either, so I decided to slip it into this cookbook, too!

In a salad bowl, toss vegetables, fruit, and beans together. Top with avocado (if using) and drizzle hot sauce (if using) and lime juice generously as a dressing.

Chef's Note Instead of hot sauce, sometimes I sprinkle cayenne or chili powder on the salad. A little sweet red chili sauce might also be delightful.

PER SERVING
WALDORF SALAD /
TROPICAL TACO SALAD

Calories 341/300
Fat. 2.4g/2g
Carbs 63.4g/65.6g
Fiber 13.4g/13.9g
Sugars. 21.4g/37.6g
Protein 15.2g/11.2g
WW Points. 8/8

SERVES 2

1 apple, cored and chopped

1–2 celery stalks, sliced

15 oz chickpeas, drained and rinsed

1 c grapes, sliced

2–3 tbsp plain vegan yogurt, unsweetened

1 head lettuce, chopped

SINGLE SERVING

4 c chopped lettuce

1 mango, peeled, seeded, and cubed

1 tomato, diced

2 green onions, sliced

½ c cooked black beans

¼ avocado (optional)

hot sauce (optional)

lime juice

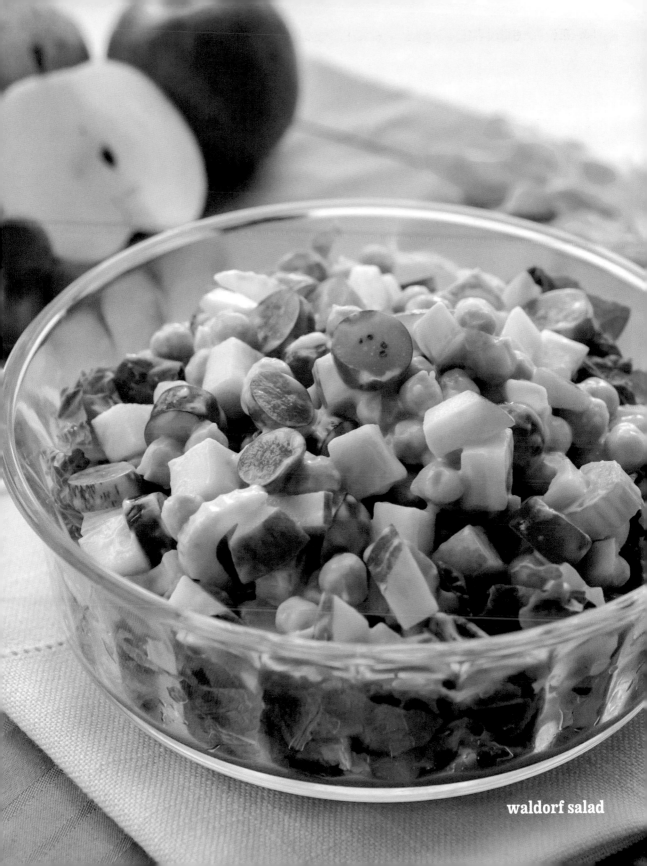

waldorf salad

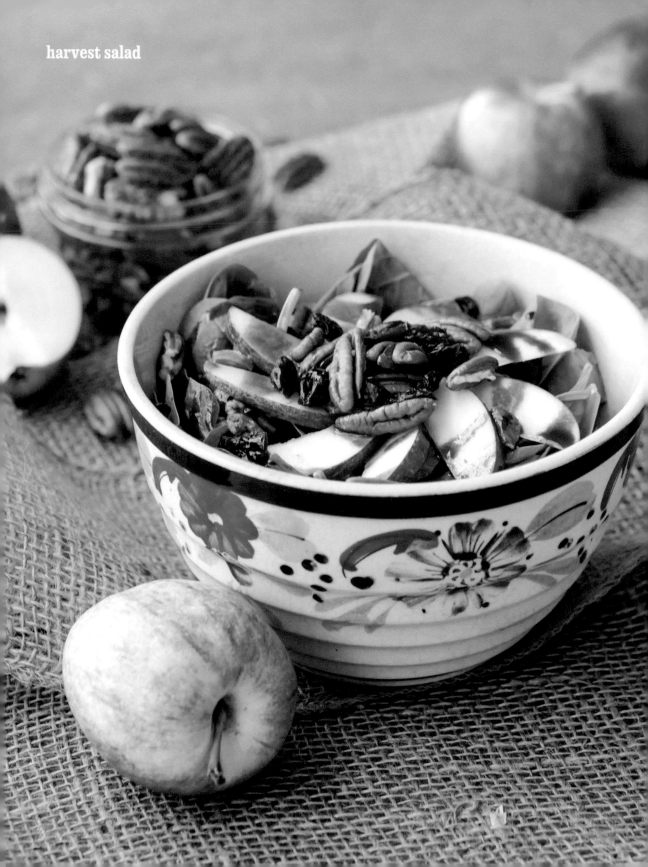

harvest salad

harvest salad

Keeping it seasonal, I started making this salad in the cooler months when my typical salad ingredients (e.g., tomatoes) start disappearing at the farmer's market.

Cook sweet potato (oven roasting is best, but micro-waving, steaming, boiling, etc. also work) and dice. Toss warm sweet potato with cold greens, apple or pear, nuts (if using), and raisins or cranberries. Drizzle Maple Vinaigrette over top and enjoy!

bbq salad

Barbecue sauce is my favorite salad dressing. It may be a little unconventional, but that's why I like it. Here's my sweet-to-heat take on a classic salad with plenty of smoky barbecue flavor to spice things up.

Toss chickpeas with barbecue sauce until well coated and briefly set aside. Place spinach in a bowl. Top with chickpeas and remaining ingredients.

PER SALAD
HARVEST SALAD WITHOUT DRESSING / BBQ SALAD

Calories 205/211
Fat. 0.7g/1.5g
Carbs 47.7g/37.8g
Fiber , ... 8.9g/7.2g
Sugars. 22.7g/6.6g
Protein 6.0g/10.1g
WW Points 7/5

SINGLE SERVING

1 sweet potato
4 c spinach or other salad greens
½ apple or pear, sliced
   walnuts or pecans (optional)
1–2 tbsp raisins or cranberries
   Maple Vinaigrette (pg. 140)

SINGLE SERVING

½ c chickpeas
1–2 tbsp barbecue sauce
2 c baby spinach
1 tsp minced fresh jalapeño (optional)
¼ c finely diced red onion
¼ c sweet corn (thawed, if using frozen)
   cilantro (optional)

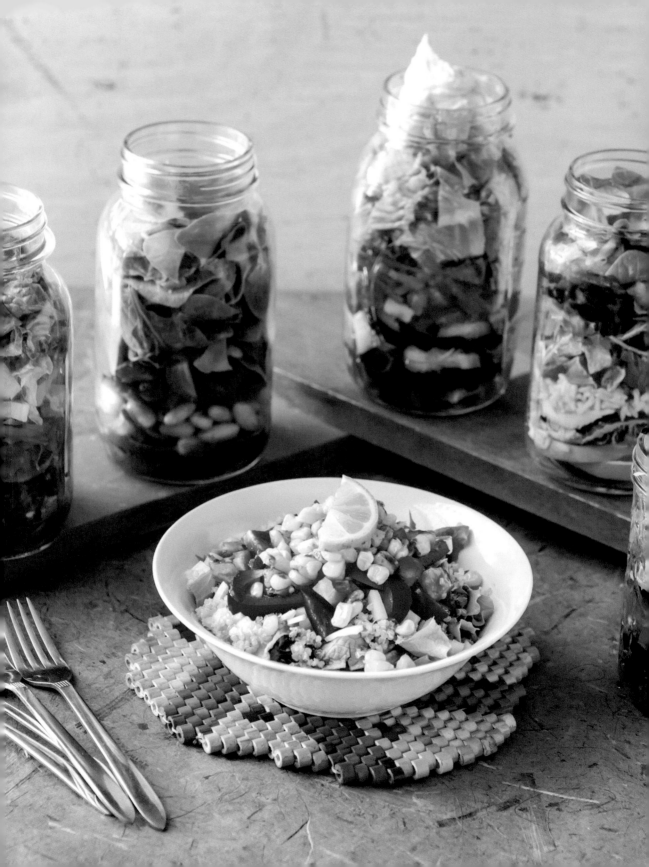

SALAD IN A JAR

Salads in mason jars are stunning (and fun!) but also a great way to take your salad to work. To make one, put your dressing in first, then your toppings, and end with your lettuce, spinach, or mixed greens (which should be the bulk of the jar—at least half). You basically assemble a salad in a jar backward compared to how you create a salad in a bowl. Chill until you're ready to eat, then dump the contents out on a plate.

You can make these ahead for the workweek and I also keep one or two in the fridge so they're there if I need a fast snack or if I need to grab one on my way out the door, ensuring I have a nutritious meal with me.

Tip: Pack your ingredients pretty well. Not so tight that you'll have trouble getting the contents back out, but you don't want a lot of extra space in the jar. Condensation will find its way into those open spaces and might make some of your vegetables soggy. Also, use the bigger, 32-oz mason jars for a meal and the smaller, 12-oz jars for snacks and side salads. Mason jars are available at most supermarkets, Target, and Walmart.

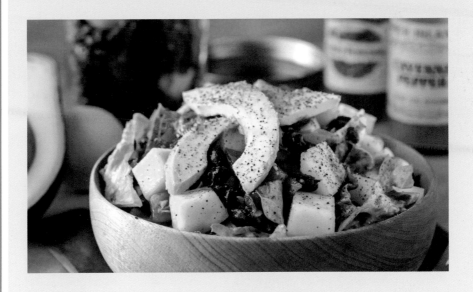

7 IDEAS FOR SALADS IN A JAR

Lindsay's fave: Balsamic-Dijon Vinaigrette (*opposite page*) or a raspberry vinaigrette, red bell pepper, green onion, chickpeas, cooked sweet potato, and baby spinach.

Basic: Italian Dressing (*opposite page*) or Balsamic-Dijon Vinaigrette (*opposite page*), red onion, cucumber, tomato, carrot, and lettuce.

Classic: Balsamic-Dijon Vinaigrette (*opposite page*), red onion, white beans, strawberries, and baby spinach.

Citrus Twist: Orange juice, orange slices, red onion, cooked barley or brown rice, sweet potato, roasted beets, and spring mix or baby spinach.

Southwest: Salsa, green onion, bell pepper, black beans, tomatoes, and lettuce.

Hummus: Bell pepper, black olives, cucumber, tomato, carrot, lettuce, and hummus on top (not at the bottom).

Zesty: Lime juice and hot sauce, corn, bell pepper, tomato, onion, cooked quinoa, and lettuce.

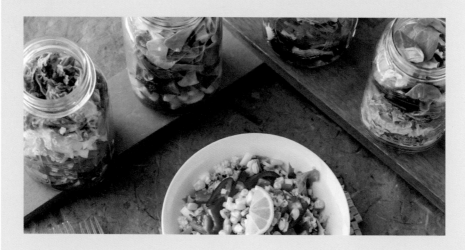

DRESSINGS TO TRY

Here are two great dressings from *Everyday Happy Herbivore* for three of the salads in a jar. For both, simply whisk all of the ingredients together, adding as much or as little agave nectar or other sweetener as needed for your level of preferred sweetness.

✔ SOY-FREE ✔ GLUTEN-FREE ✔ FAT-FREE ✔ QUICK ✔ BUDGET ✔ PANTRY ✔ SINGLE SERVING

Balsamic-Dijon Vinaigrette

2 tsp Dijon mustard
1 tsp balsamic vinegar
1 tsp red wine vinegar
1 tbsp water
   agave nectar (or other sweetener) to taste

> Calories 1; Fat 1.7g; Total Carbs 17.4g; Fiber 6g; Sugars 7.6g; Protein 10.4g; WW Points 1

Italian Dressing

2 tbsp apple cider vinegar*
¼ tsp Dijon mustard
   several dashes of Italian seasoning
   dash of onion powder
   dash of garlic powder
   agave nectar (or other sweetener) to taste

> Calories 11; Fat 0.2g; Total Carbs 0.9g; Fiber 0g; Sugars 0g; Protein 0.1g; WW Points 1

* If you like, you can substitute other vinegars, such as distilled white vinegar or red wine vinegar.

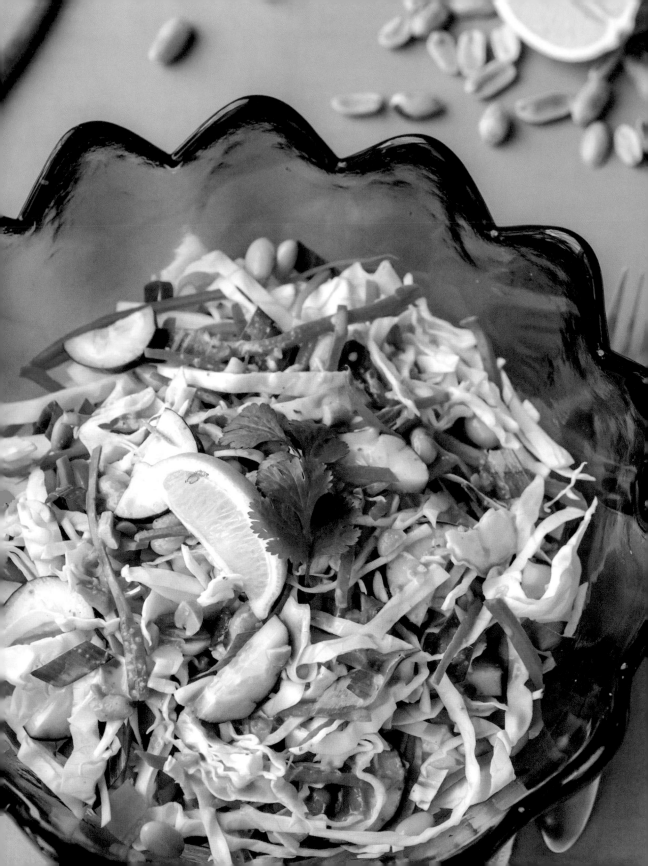

thai crunch

Before I was plant-based, I loved the Thai Crunch salad at California Pizza Kitchen. I finally decided to re-create a lighter vegan version of it for this cookbook. It's easy, fresh, fast, and satisfying. (I also loved their Original BBQ Chicken Chopped salad, hence *my* BBQ Salad [pg. 133] recipe!) By the way, CPK is one of the vegan-friendliest restaurant chains in the US. They have a PDF online indicating which menu items are suitable for vegans and vegetarians.

Toss cabbage/lettuce, carrot, green onions, edamame, and cucumber together in a salad bowl, then top with Thai Peanut Dressing, crushed peanuts, and cilantro (if using), and garnish with a lime wedge. (I also love squeezing fresh lime juice over the salad.)

PER SERVING

Calories	300
Fat	11.7g
Carbs	39.4g
Fiber	13.7g
Sugars	16.3g
Fat	17.3g
WW Points	8

SINGLE SERVING

- 4 c napa cabbage, red cabbage, or lettuce (or a combination)
- 1 carrot, julienned
- 2 green onions, sliced
- ¼ –½ c edamame
- ½ cucumber, sliced or diced
- Thai Peanut Dressing (pg. 140)
- crushed peanuts (optional garnish)
- cilantro (optional)
- lime wedges (garnish)

Chef's Note For a soy-free version, substitute chickpeas for the edamame.

☒☒ THE BEST

thai peanut dressing

Creamy, delicious—here's a lower fat and lower calorie DIY peanut sauce.

MAKES ¼ CUP

- 1 tbsp smooth peanut butter
- 1 tbsp warm water
- 1 tbsp sweet red chili sauce
- juice of 1 lime wedge
- 2 tsp low-sodium soy sauce or gluten-free tamari
- 1¼ tsp rice vinegar
- garlic powder
- ground ginger
- 1–2 drops Asian hot sauce (e.g., Sriracha)
- 1 tbsp nondairy milk

In a small, microwave-safe bowl, add peanut butter with water, chili sauce, lime juice, soy sauce or tamari, rice vinegar, a few dashes of garlic powder and ground ginger, plus hot sauce. Microwave for 10–20 seconds (so peanut butter is melty), whisk into a sauce, and then whisk in nondairy milk. Taste, adding more hot sauce as desired.

Chef's Note For a richer sauce, substitute coconut milk for the nondairy.

maple vinaigrette

MAKES 2½ TBSP

- 1 tbsp pure maple syrup
- 1 tbsp balsamic vinegar
- 1– 1½ tsp Dijon mustard
- dash of ground ginger

Whisk ingredients together. Taste, adding more Dijon if desired.

golden dressing

My friend Chef AJ turned me on to the miso-mustard-nutritional-yeast combination and I've been playing with it ever since. What I love most about this dressing is that you can make small adjustments and have a whole new flavor. For example, add more miso for a miso dressing. More Dijon for a spicy or tangy dressing, more lemon, and so on. I also like to substitute peanut butter for the miso on occasion.

Combine all ingredients in a blender and blend until smooth and creamy, adding more water if you like a thinner dressing (note: this dressing thickens as it chills in the fridge). Taste, adding more nutritional yeast, Dijon, maple, lemon, or miso as desired.

PER SERVING
WITH MISO/WITH PEANUT BUTTER
(1 TSP EACH)

Calories	21/25
Fat	0.3g/0.9g
Carbs	3.3g/3.2g
Fiber	1g/1g
Sugars	1.2g/1.2g
Protein	1.8g/1.9g
WW Points	1

MAKES ABOUT ½ CUP

- ¼ c cold water
- ¼ c nutritional yeast
- 1–2 tbsp Dijon mustard
- 1 tbsp pure maple syrup or 1–2 dates
- ½ lemon, skin removed and seeded
- 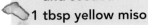 1 tbsp yellow miso

Chef's Note I use yellow miso, but white or red should also work. Do not use brown miso.

PER SERVING

Calories 257
Fat 2.3g
Carbs 56.9g
Fiber 5.6g
Sugars 31.1g
Protein 5.5g
WW Points 7

SINGLE SERVING

- 1 c cubed mango
- ½ c cooked quinoa (warm or chilled)
- 1 green onion, sliced
- ¼ c cilantro
- 1–2 tbsp sweet red chili sauce
- juice of 2 lime wedges

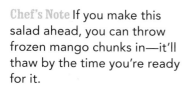

Chef's Note If you make this salad ahead, you can throw frozen mango chunks in—it'll thaw by the time you're ready for it.

spicy mango quinoa salad

This is my go-to meal when I'm not quite hungry enough for a big meal but need something more substantial than a light snack to feel satisfied. I also like to serve this as a starter salad in the summer or anytime we're having sushi or spring rolls for dinner. For a more meal-sized version, serve it over a bed of spinach with cubed tofu or adzuki beans.

Combine mango, quinoa, green onion, cilantro, and 1 tbsp sweet red chili sauce in a bowl, and stir to combine. Squeeze in lime juice and mix again. Taste, adding more chili sauce as desired.

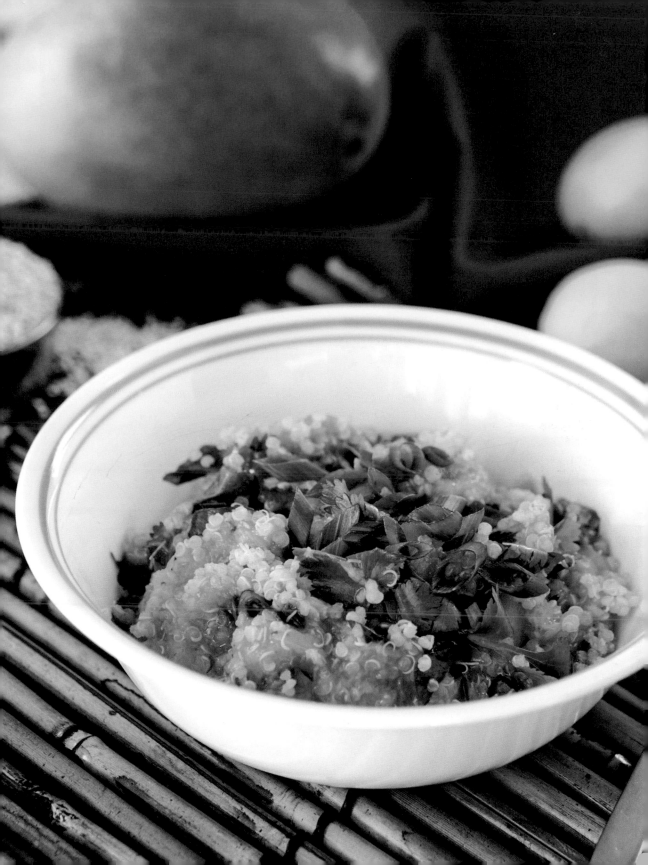

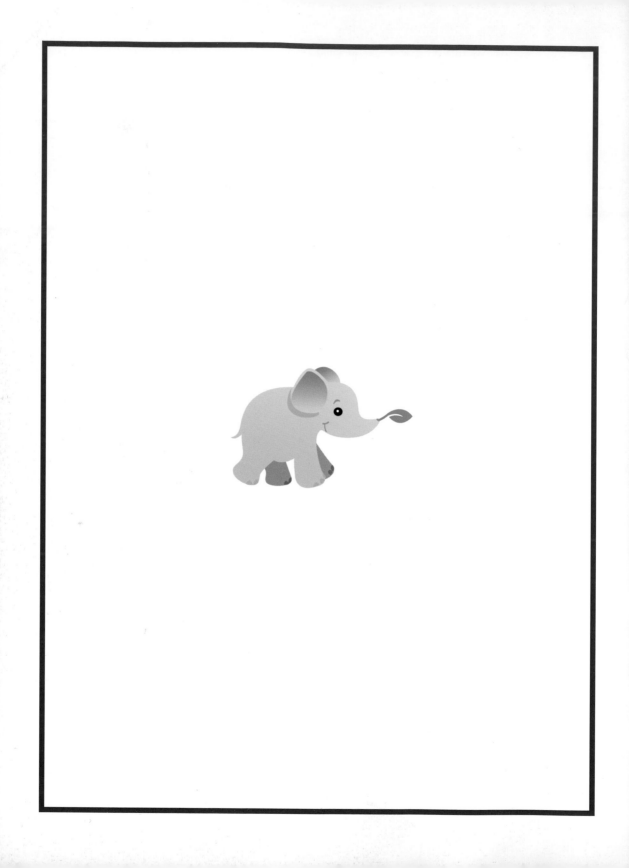

pasta, stir-fries & noodles

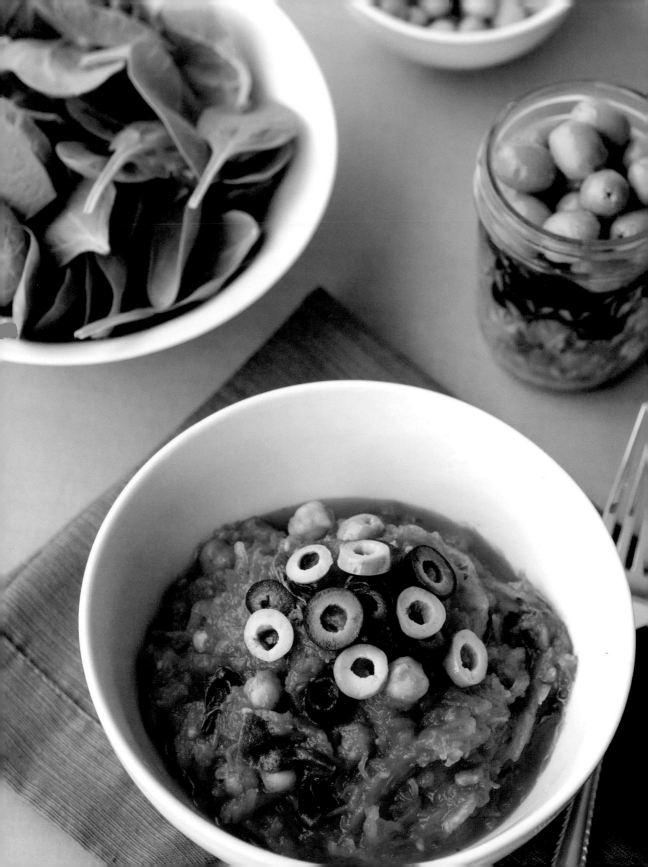

skinny puttanesca

You might remember the puttanesca in *Everyday Happy Herbivore*. This is a slimmed down version of that dish, using spaghetti squash instead of pasta. You'll be pleasantly surprised how stuffed (and satisfied!) you feel after eating this. Skinny Puttanesca is also one of the most requested dishes on my 7-Day Meal Plans!

Stab squash a few times with a fork and microwave whole for 10 minutes or until it's fork-tender. Carefully slice the squash in half and allow it to cool so it's safe to handle. Meanwhile, line a skillet with a thin layer of water or broth and sauté garlic for a minute. Then add red pepper flakes and cook another minute or two, until both are fragrant. Then add spinach and tomato, plus a splash of additional water if needed. (You can also add 1 tbsp extra marinara sauce here for more flavor.) Continue to cook, stirring constantly, until the spinach turns a darker green and the tomato softens but neither are mushy or falling apart, about 45 seconds, then set aside. Once squash is cool, spoon out seedy matter, discard, then run a fork lengthwise down the squash to remove all the "pasta" strands. Measure out 3 cups, saving the rest. Combine "pasta" with the warmed marinara until it's lightly, but evenly, coated with sauce. Plate and season with salt and pepper, if desired. Top with spinach-tomato mixture, olives, and chickpeas (if using).

PER SERVING

Calories 304
Fat 8.6g
Carbs 57.2g
Fiber 11.2g
Sugars 22.8g
Protein 11.5g
WW Points 9

SINGLE SERVING

- 3 c spaghetti squash (about ½ a medium squash)
- 2 garlic cloves, minced
- pinch red pepper flakes
- 2 c baby spinach
- 1 tomato, diced
- 1 c Marinara Sauce (pg. 263), warmed
- 6 tbsp black or green (or combination) olives
- chickpeas (optional)

Chef's Note No microwave? Cut squash in half lengthwise and bake it cut-side-down on a cookie sheet for 30–45 minutes at 350°F.

PER SERVING
(WITHOUT MARINARA SAUCE)

Calories 202
Fat. 5.5g
Carbs 33.3g
Fiber 10.4g
Sugars. 8.4g
Protein 7.6g
WW Points. 5

SERVES 4

- 2 small eggplants
- 1 c breadcrumbs (see Chef's Note)
- 4 tbsp AJ's Vegan Parmesan (pg. 271)
- 2 tbsp Italian seasoning
- ¼ tsp fine salt
- ⅛ tsp pepper
- ½ c nondairy milk
- 1 tbsp cornstarch
- 1 28-oz jar marinara sauce

Chef's Notes

» Skin is optional on the eggplant. Some people like it, some people find it too chewy.

» You can make your own breadcrumbs by toasting a piece of bread and then chopping it up into crumbs in your blender or food processor.

eggplant parm

One recipe I'm always getting a request for is eggplant Parmesan, so here's my healthy take on the classic Italian dish. When my friend Nichelle tried it, she e-mailed, "This was definitely a great guilt-free substitute to cheesy eggplant Parm, that you can feel okay with eating more often."

Slice eggplant into ¼–½-inch rounds. Rinse with water. Place a drying rack on a clean kitchen towel, then place eggplant on rack. Sprinkle with salt (coarse is best) and let rest 30 minutes (this allows the solanine, what makes eggplant bitter, to leach out). Brush off salt with a damp cloth.

Meanwhile, preheat oven to 350°F. Line a cookie sheet with parchment paper and set aside. Combine breadcrumbs, Parmesan, Italian seasoning, salt, and pepper, then finely grind in a food processor or with a mortar and pestle to a fine, sandlike consistency. Pour crumb mixture into a shallow bowl. Whisk nondairy milk and cornstarch together, then pour into another shallow bowl. Dip each eggplant round into the nondairy mixture, briefly submerging it, then immediately into the breadcrumbs mixture. Flip eggplant over and press into the breadcrumbs again, repeating as necessary so it is well coated. Repeat with remaining eggplant slices, placing the finished product on the cookie sheet. Bake for 12 minutes. Flip them over and bake

TEN TIPS FOR SCRIMPING ON CALORIES

1. Brush your teeth between meals.

2. Drink a glass of water before eating.

3. Place a celery stalk front and center in your fridge. If you're truly hungry, you'll eat it. If you're pushing your hand past it, chances are something else is at play.

4. When eating out, order a large salad (with lemon juice or hot sauce in place of dressing) and eat it first, before your entrée.

5. Use smaller plates and bowls. A little food on a big plate sets you up for feeling deprived. Food spilling out on a small plate makes you feel like nothing is limited.

6. Think in color. Eat lots of color.

7. Keep serving bowls off the table. You have to get up and walk somewhere else for seconds.

8. Put a napkin on your plate as soon as you're done eating, especially when eating out, so you don't continue to nibble waiting for everyone else to finish or the waiter to come by.

9. CHEW.

10. Lighten up a meal by serving it over greens instead of grains.

for 5–10 minutes more. If necessary, bake another 5–10 minutes, flipping them halfway through. Bake until eggplant is soft and crumbs have taken on a deeper, more golden coloring—but be careful not to burn (time may vary based on how thick your slices are).

Arrange eggplant slices on a plate, cover with marinara sauce, and garnish with vegan Parmesan.

skinny mac 'n' cheese

PER SERVING

Calories 131
Fat 2.1g
Carbs 21.4g
Fiber 5.3g
Sugars 1.5g
Protein 9.5g
WW Points 3

SERVES 4

"CHEESE" SAUCE

1 c nondairy milk

⅓ c nutritional yeast

2 tbsp tomato sauce or ketchup

1 tbsp cornstarch

½ tsp onion powder

½ tsp garlic powder

½ c pure pumpkin (canned)

2 c cooked whole-wheat or gluten-free pasta

4 c chopped greens (e.g., spinach or kale)

hot sauce (optional)

I stumbled across a "diet" macaroni and cheese in a magazine that combined butternut squash with low-fat cheese to cut calories. I decided to nix the cheese (and the butternut) and slip a little pumpkin into my classic Easy Macaroni and Cheese recipe—just to see what it would taste like. Winner! Winner! Chickpea dinner! Dare I say I like this "lighter" squashy version better than the original? To extend this dish further, add cubed (and cooked) butternut squash or sweet potato and double the sauce.

In a small saucepan, whisk all "cheese" sauce ingredients together and heat over low, stirring regularly, until it's warm and thick. Season with salt and pepper if desired.

Meanwhile, bring a pot of water to a boil and add pasta. Cook until al dente (according to package instructions; it varies). Just before the pasta is done cooking (about a minute before) add in greens, and stir constantly until greens get darker in color and soften, but aren't completely mush (time varies depending on greens used). Drain pasta and greens and return to pot. Add "cheese" sauce over top and stir to combine. Spoon into bowls and drizzle generously with hot sauce if using.

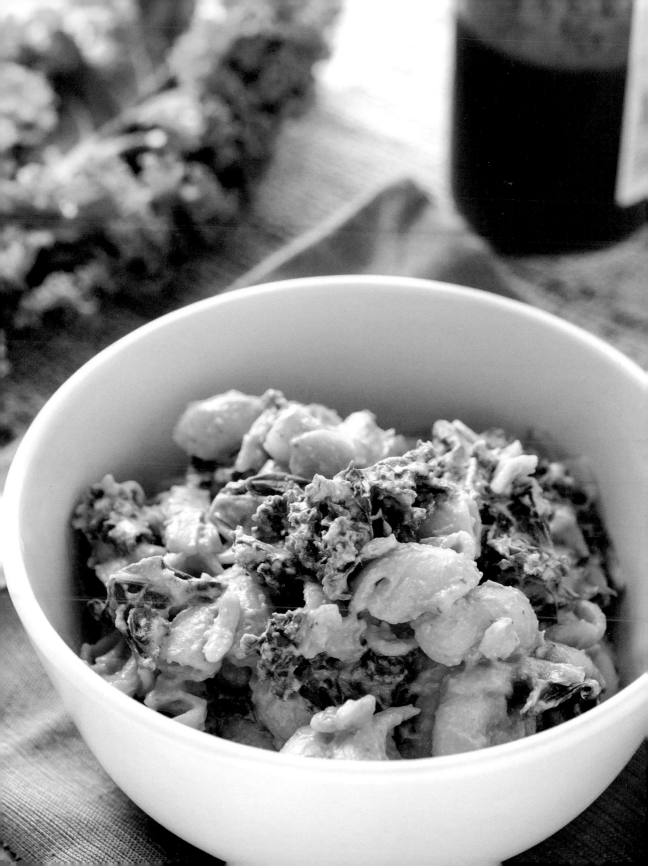

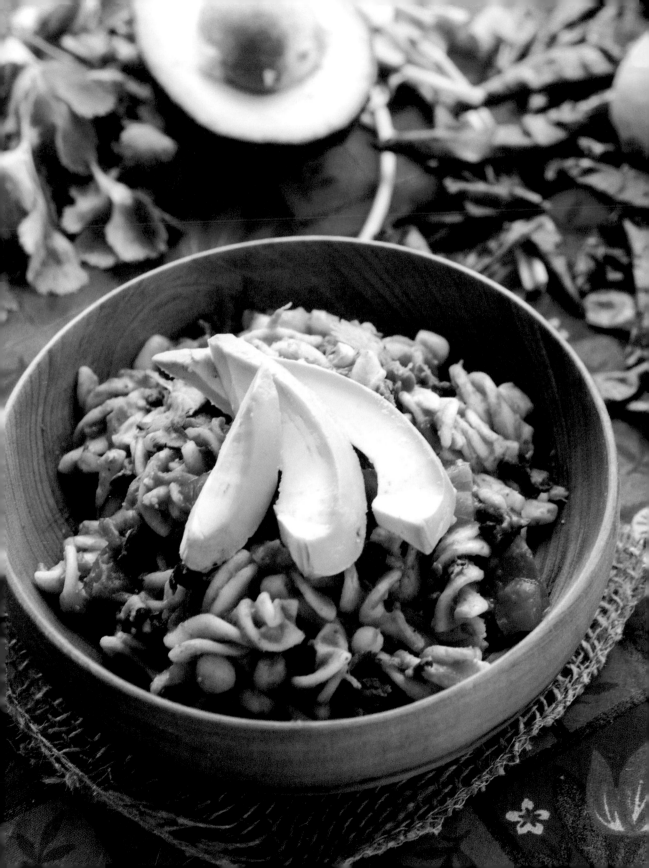

chipotle pasta

Don't be put off by the long list of ingredients; this recipe comes together quickly and is relatively effortless. Just stir, heat, dump—go! It's the sassy sister to mac 'n' cheese, with healthy additions like beans, corn, and tomato slipped in.

Cook pasta according to package instructions, adding the corn and beans in the last minute or so to warm them up, then drain. Meanwhile, whisk all sauce ingredients together (except lime juice), starting with ¼ cup salsa and ¼ tsp chipotle powder and bring to a boil, stirring constantly. Once boiling, reduce heat to low and continue to cook until the sauce has thickened. Taste, adding more salsa or chipotle as desired, keeping in mind that a little goes a long way. You can also add cayenne to taste for an even hotter sauce. Turn off heat and stir in lime juice, plus salt to taste if desired. Pour over pasta/corn/bean mixture, and stir to coat. Stir in tomatoes, plus avocado and cilantro if using.

Chef's Notes

» Kidney beans or pinto beans may be substituted for the black beans

» For a gluten-free version, use gluten-free pasta and gluten-free flour in the sauce.

PER SERVING
(WITHOUT AVOCADO)

Calories	152
Fat	2.2g
Carbs	25.1g
Fiber	7.4g
Sugars	2.3g
Protein	10.4g
WW Points	4

SERVES 4

- 8 oz whole-wheat pasta
- 1 c corn
- 1 15-oz can black beans, drained and rinsed
- 1 tomato, diced
- 1 avocado, diced (optional)
- cilantro (optional)

SAUCE

- ¼ –½ c salsa
- ¼ –½ tsp chipotle powder
- 1 c nondairy milk
- ⅓ c nutritional yeast
- 2 tbsp white whole-wheat flour
- 1 tbsp yellow miso
- 1 tsp onion powder
- ½ tsp garlic powder
- ½ tsp ground cumin
- ¼ c tomato sauce
- 2 tbsp minced green chilies (canned)
- 1 tsp lime juice

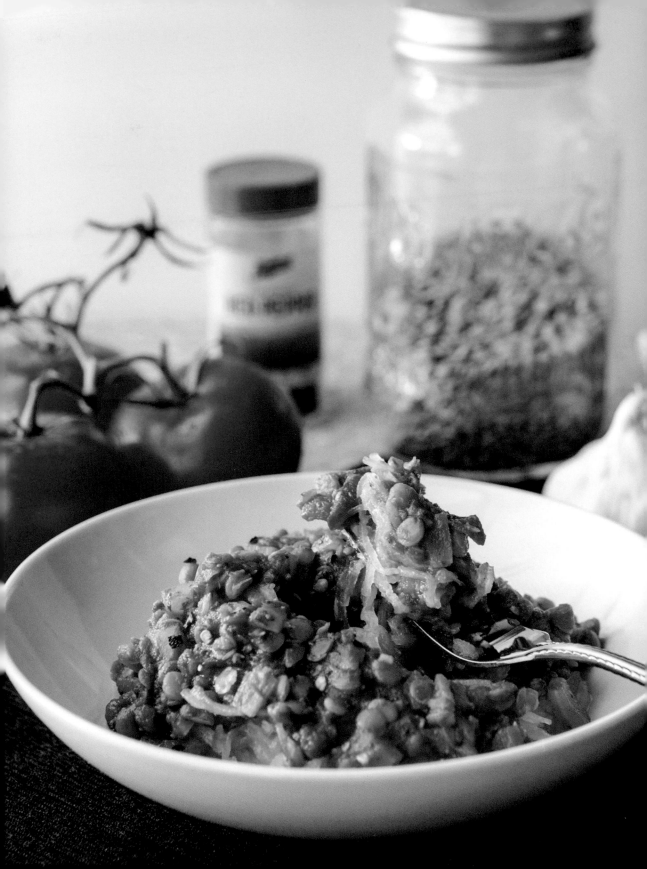

lentil marinara sauce

This hearty marinara is crazy filling and scratches that pasta itch. I like to serve it over spaghetti squash for a lower calorie "spaghetti" experience, but it's great on baked potatoes, broccoli, or anything you'd usually smother with marinara sauce. By the way, the flavor intensifies over time, so make ahead if you can and look forward to leftovers!

Line a medium pot with a thin layer of broth and sauté garlic and onion over high heat until onion is translucent, about 2 minutes. Add required remaining ingredients (starting with 2 tbsp tomato paste) and bring to a boil. Once boiling, reduce heat to low, and simmer until lentils are soft and cooked, about 20–30 minutes. Allow to cool so it's not lava hot and taste, adding more tomato paste if desired, plus salt and pepper. If it's too acidic, you can add a pinch of sugar or a quick squeeze of ketchup. If it's not saucy enough for you, add more broth or tomato sauce to thin it out.

PER SERVING
(1 CUP)

Calories	133
Fat	1.7g
Carbs	21.6g
Fiber	8.4g
Sugars	6.5g
Protein	8.6g
WW Points	3

MAKES 5 CUPS

- 2 c vegetable broth, divided
- 3–4 garlic cloves, minced
- 1 small onion, diced
- 2–3 tbsp tomato paste
- 2 tomatoes, diced (optional)
- 1 15-oz can diced tomatoes
- 1 tbsp Italian seasoning
- 1 tbsp red wine vinegar
- ½ c red lentils
- 1 small jalapeño, chopped, stem discarded
- sugar or ketchup (optional)

Chef's Note If desired, you can transfer part (or all) of the sauce to a blender and blend until smooth (I like it chunky). Fire-roasted tomatoes—instead of plain diced—also add a little something extra to this dish.

PER SERVING
(1 TBSP)/ENTIRE RECIPE

Calories 9/117
Fat. 0.1g/1.2g
Carbs 2g/22.6g
Fiber. 0g/7.6g
Sugars. 1.1g/14.5g
Protein 0.5g/4.3g
WW Points. 0

MAKES 1 CUP

- 1 12-oz jar roasted red peppers (in water, not oil), drained (about 3 peppers)
- 1 c fresh basil (packed tight)
- 1–2 garlic cloves
- 1 tsp fresh lemon juice

red pesto

Why does green pesto get to have all the fun? This red pesto combines basil with roasted red peppers and whips up in seconds! Use it in any way you'd use pesto: as a spread, tossed with pasta, and so on.

Combine all ingredients in a blender or small food processor and whiz until smooth. Add a tiny splash of water or vegetable broth if necessary, but avoid it so the pesto doesn't get too wet or watery. Taste, adding more basil as desired, plus salt and pepper.

Chef's Note When serving this as an appetizer spread on crusty bread, I garnish with a little vegan Parmesan.

The easiest way to cut back on calories in stir-fries is to remove the "fry" part—take out the oil. You can also cut the fat and calories by using nondairy milk to replace all or part of the coconut milk (just add a drop or two of coconut extract!).

cream sauce

This protein-packed cream sauce is perfect for pasta or as a dip for crusty bread. I also like to smother veggies with it—favorites include peas and broccoli. Use this sauce any way you'd use an Alfredo (even though it doesn't taste *exactly* like an Alfredo sauce). It's crazy easy and addictive!

Combine all ingredients from chickpeas through vegan Parmesan in a blender or mini food processor, and puree until smooth and creamy (and runny like Alfredo; it shouldn't be thick like hummus). Transfer to a saucepan and warm over low heat, stirring often until thoroughly warm. Once warm, add a little bit of fresh lemon juice (a slight squeeze), and stir to combine. Taste, adding more lemon or more vegan Parmesan if desired. Add a dash of smoked paprika for a smoked flavor (a little goes a long way). I also like to sprinkle black pepper over top before serving.

PER SERVING
(1¼ CUPS)

Calories	189
Fat	2.1g
Carbs	30.5g
Fiber	11.5g
Sugars	2.8g
Protein	14g
WW Points	4

MAKES 1¼ CUPS

⅓ c cooked chickpeas
⅔ c cooked white beans
1 tsp yellow miso
½ tsp garlic powder
½ tsp onion powder
   dash ground nutmeg
½ c nondairy milk
¼ c nutritional yeast
2–3 tbsp vegan Parmesan
   juice of 1 lemon wedge
   smoked paprika

Chef's Note Any white bean, such as navy, butter, or cannellini, will work here.

soba peanut noodles

PER SERVING

Calories	274
Fat	6g
Carbs	47.5g
Fiber	6.6g
Sugars	6.7g
Protein	10.4g
WW Points	7

SERVES 2

- 4 oz buckwheat noodles (could sub spaghetti)
- 2 green onions, sliced
- cubed tofu or edamame (optional)
- vegetables, like broccoli or cucumber (optional)

CREAMY PEANUT SAUCE

- 2 tbsp plain vegan yogurt
- 1 tbsp smooth peanut butter
- 1 tbsp sweet red chili sauce
- few dashes garlic powder
- few dashes ground ginger
- 1 tbsp rice vinegar
- 1–2 tsp low-sodium soy sauce or gluten-free tamari
- Asian hot sauce (e.g., Sriracha; optional)

All the taste you love in creamy peanut noodles but with less fat and calories thanks to a surprise ingredient: vegan yogurt! I call this a "cheater" recipe since I use a dab of peanut butter, but it's still light compared to most peanut noodle recipes.

Cook noodles according to package instructions, rinse under cold water in a colander, and chill in the fridge for a few minutes if you can. Meanwhile, whisk peanut sauce ingredients together. Taste, adding more soy sauce or tamari, garlic, onion, or hot sauce as desired. Toss noodles with sauce, then stir in green onion, tofu or edamame if using, and vegetables, if using.

Chef's Note Despite having "wheat" in the name, buckwheat flour is completely gluten-free. Just make sure your noodles are 100% buckwheat if you have an allergy or sensitivity.

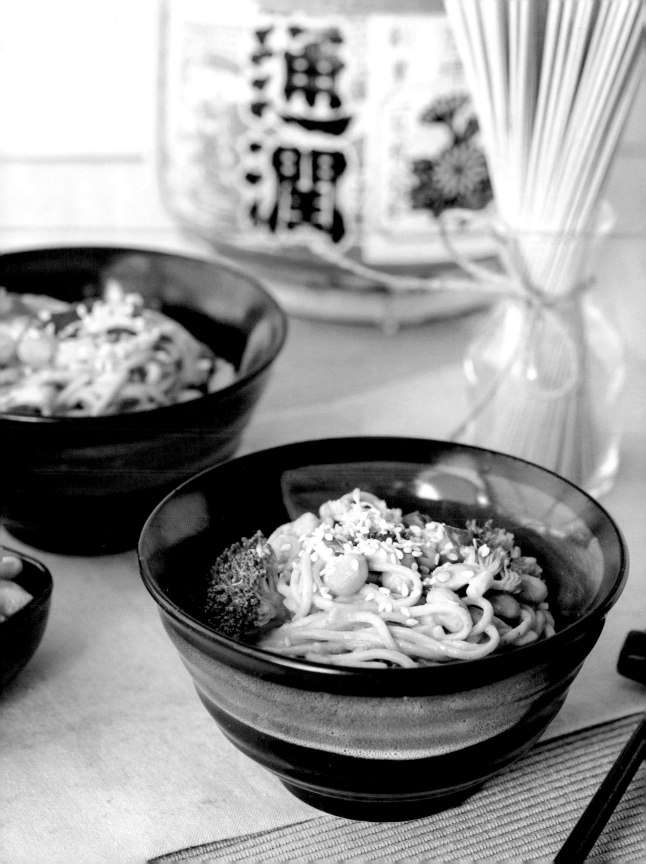

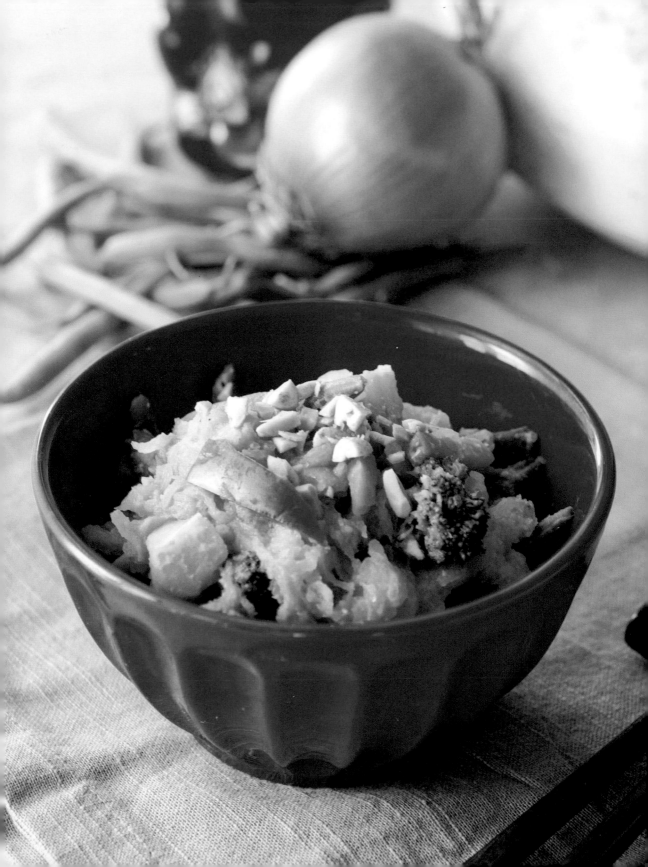

skinny pad thai

My "Cheater" Pad Thai recipe from *The Happy Herbivore Cookbook* is, hands down, one of my most popular recipes. It may even be the *most* popular. I wanted to create a lighter version of that recipe for this cookbook. (Plus, how else would you use up the leftover spaghetti squash from the Skinny Puttanesca [pg. 147]?) For a more filling meal, add cubed tofu. Sliced green onion and crushed peanuts also make a great garnish. For a spicy kick, drizzle some Sriracha!

Stab spaghetti squash a few times with a fork and microwave it whole for about 10 minutes, or until it's fork-tender. Carefully slice the squash in half and allow it to cool so it's safe to handle. Meanwhile, cook veggies according to package instructions and in a small bowl whisk 2 tbsp of warm water, soy sauce or tamari, peanut butter, chili sauce, garlic powder, ground ginger, and hot sauce together until combined. It may appear too runny at first, but it's not. Taste, adding more hot sauce if desired. Once squash is cool, spoon out seedy matter and discard, then run a fork lengthwise down the squash to remove all the "pasta" strands. Measure out 3 cups, saving the rest. Combine "pasta" with the Pad Thai Sauce until it's lightly but evenly coated with sauce. Stir in vegetables, garnish, and serve.

PER SERVING

Calories	296
Fat	9.8g
Carbs	45.8g
Fiber	6.7g
Sugars	11.6g
Protein	10.8g
WW Points	8

SINGLE SERVING

- 3 c spaghetti squash (about ½ a medium squash)
- 7 oz frozen stir-fry mixed vegetables

PAD THAI SAUCE

- 2 tbsp warm water
- 2 tbsp low-sodium soy sauce or gluten-free tamari
- 1 tbsp smooth peanut butter
- 1 tbsp sweet red chili Asian sauce
- ¼ tsp granulated garlic powder
- ¼ tsp ground ginger
- ¼ tsp hot sauce, or to taste

Chef's Note No microwave? Cut squash in half lengthwise and bake it cut-side down on a cookie sheet for 30–45 minutes at 350°F.

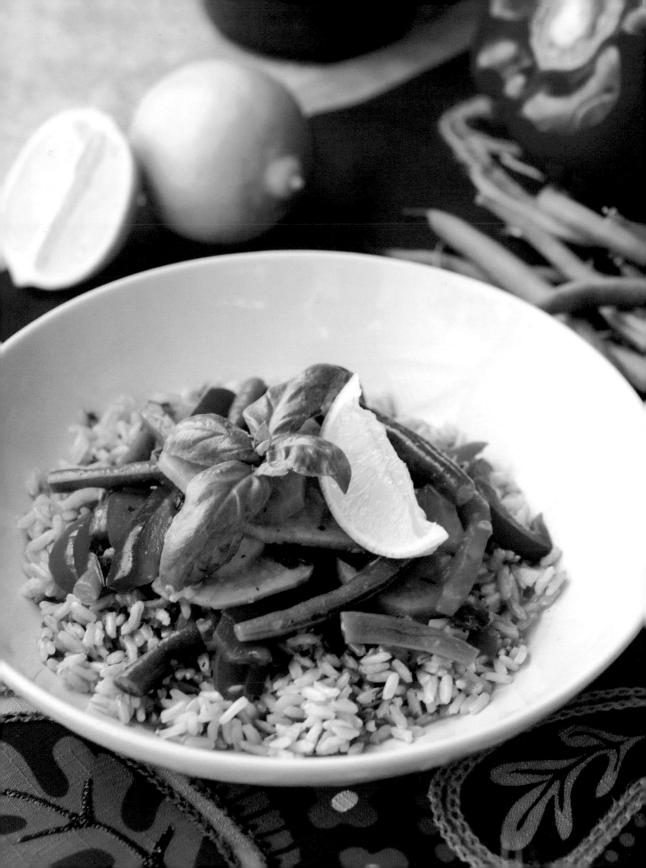

bangkok curry

String beans and sweet potatoes show up in this Thai delight, creating a new stir-fry experience. For a fuller meal, add cubed tofu and serve over brown rice.

Trim green beans and cut in half if they are long; set aside. Slice sweet potato into ⅛–¼-inch thick rounds, or cube, and set aside. Line a large skillet with a thin layer of broth and sauté ginger, garlic, green onions (reserving some dark green parts for garnish), and a dash or pinch of red pepper flakes, if using, until water has evaporated and garlic is golden, about a minute. Add more broth to line the bottom, plus the green beans, sweet potato slices, bell pepper, and 1 tsp curry powder, stirring to combine and coat veggies. Cover, bring to a boil, then reduce heat to medium and simmer until potatoes are fork-tender and pepper soft, but still crisp, about 3 minutes (add splashes of broth if necessary). Add coconut milk, soy sauce or tamari, and sweet red chili sauce, and stir. Taste, adding more curry if desired. Heat for about a minute over low, then add basil and stir. Heat for another minute (until thoroughly warm) and add green onion and lime wedge garnish.

Chef's Notes

» For a lower-fat version, use nondairy milk with a drop or two of coconut extract instead of coconut milk.

» If you want to use frozen green beans, add them at the end and cook for another minute or so until they are warm, but still crisp.

PER SERVING

Calories	119
Fat	4.8g
Carbs	18.3g
Fiber	2.9g
Sugars	6.6g
Protein	2.6g
WW Points	3

SERVES 2

- 1 c green beans
- 1 sweet potato, peeled and sliced or diced
- ½ c low-sodium vegetable broth
- 1 tbsp minced fresh ginger
- 2–3 garlic cloves, minced
- 2 green onions, sliced
- dash red pepper flakes (optional)
- 1 red bell pepper, seeded and sliced
- 1– 1½ tsp mild yellow curry powder
- 1 c light coconut milk
- 1 tsp low-sodium soy sauce or gluten-free tamari
- 1 tbsp sweet red chili sauce
- 1–2 tbsp fresh basil, minced
- lime wedges (garnish)

UNDER
150
CALORIES

Nom Nom!
6/2014

thai green curry

A slimmed-down version of the classic Thai dish. It whips together fast and always hits the spot when you want Thai takeout. Serve over brown rice.

PER SERVING

Calories 111
Fat 5.3g
Carbs 14.1g
Fiber 0.6g
Sugars 4.7g
Protein 2.4g
WW Points 3

SERVES 2

- 8 oz frozen stir-fry mixed vegetables
- ½ c nondairy milk
- ½ c light coconut milk
- 1 tbsp green curry paste (I use Thai Kitchen)
- 1 tbsp low-sodium soy sauce or gluten-free tamari
- 1 tbsp brown sugar
- ¼ tsp ground ginger (powder, not fresh)
  fresh basil
- 1 green onion, sliced

Chef's Note Soy milk works best in this recipe (for the nondairy milk).

Place frozen vegetables in a skillet and heat over high. Add a tiny bit of broth or water if you want, but you shouldn't need any—as the frozen vegetables thaw, they release some liquid. Meanwhile, whisk milks, curry paste, soy sauce or tamari, sugar, and ground ginger together. As soon as vegetables are almost cooked, add sauce, and reduce heat to low. Then add basil (about a handful, ¼ cup or so—it's okay to be generous; I have used eight large leaves and could have added more) and green onion. Stir to combine and heat until totally warm and basil has wilted and softened, about 2–3 minutes. Taste, adding more curry paste, soy sauce or tamari, ground ginger, or sugar if desired. The longer you let it sit, the more the basil will flavor the sauce. I always like to let it cool for a few minutes before serving.

add lime juice (1 lime)
shredded coconut
top c cashews

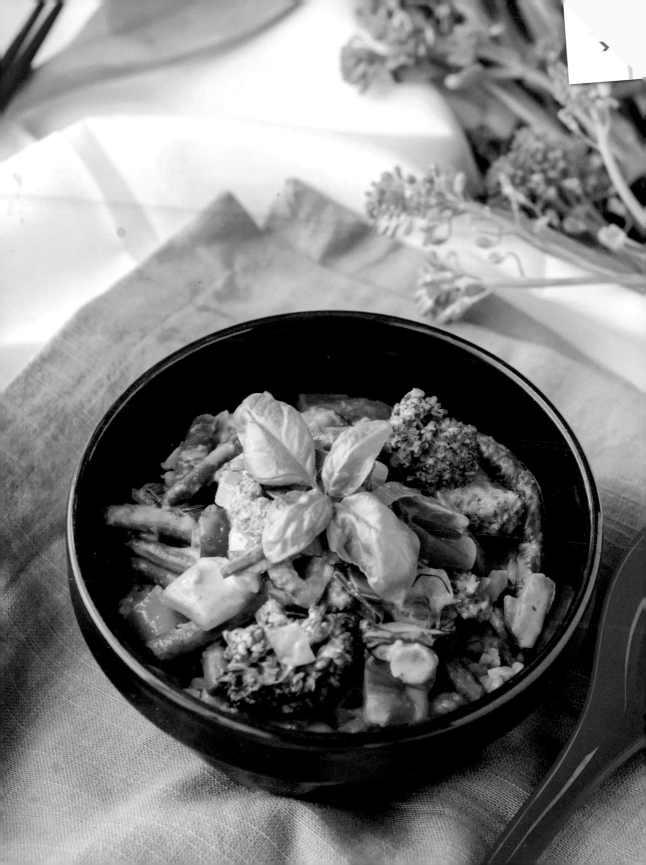

PER SERVING
(½ CUP)

Calories	78
Fat	0.7g
Carbs	16.8g
Fiber	2.4g
Sugars	5.6g
Protein	1.7g
WW Points	2

MAKES 2 CUPS

- 2 green onions, sliced
- ¾ c low-sodium vegetable broth, divided
- 4 garlic cloves, minced
- 1 tbsp minced fresh ginger
- 2 small sweet potatoes, peeled and diced
- ½ c nondairy milk
- 2 tsp brown sugar
- ¼ –1 tsp red curry paste (I use Thai Kitchen)
- low-sodium soy sauce or gluten-free tamari (optional)
- juice of lime wedges
- cilantro (garnish)

Chef's Note You can mix a little peanut butter in (to taste) for a peanut-flavored curry.

thai sweet potato curry sauce

This easy curry has just the right creamy consistency and sweet-to-heat ratio I love about Thai vegetable dishes but without all the fatty coconut milk. I like to serve this sauce with cooked bell pepper strips and diced tofu over a bed of brown rice, but other veggies work, too.

Set aside a few dark green onion pieces for garnish. Line a saucepan with a thin layer of broth and sauté onion, garlic, and ginger over high heat for a minute or two, until fragrant and garlic is golden. Add sweet potatoes and additional broth if necessary, so a thin layer of liquid lines the pot. Cover, bring to a boil, and simmer 5–10 minutes until sweet potatoes are tender, but not overcooked and mushy. Transfer mixture to a blender and add ½ cup broth, ½ cup nondairy milk, brown sugar, ¼ tsp red curry paste, and whiz until smooth and creamy, adding more broth if necessary. Return to saucepan and heat over low. Taste, whisking in more red curry paste as desired. Season with low-sodium soy sauce or tamari if desired. Add fresh lime juice just before serving and garnish with reserved green onion and cilantro.

ginger cabbage stir-fry

My friend Kael ordered a ginger-tempeh stir-fry at Real Food Daily in Los Angeles that was incredible. It was one of those dishes that I'd scanned past a dozen times and never would have ordered for myself but after tasting some of his, I was sorry I hadn't. I set out to re-create that meal and ended up with this filling dish. To bulk up the dish, serve over brown rice or stir in noodles such as soba noodles.

In a large pot, add hot sauce (if using), jalapeño, red onion, ginger, 1 tbsp soy sauce or tamari, 1 tbsp rice vinegar, garlic, and ¼ cup (4 tbsp) pineapple juice, and stir to combine. Sauté over high heat for a minute or two, then add tempeh and continue to cook for another minute. Add cornstarch slurry, reduce heat to medium, and allow mixture to thicken into a glaze. Reduce heat to low, stir in cabbage (it will soften a bit), and add remaining 1 tbsp soy sauce or tamari, 1 tbsp rice vinegar, and 2 tbsp hot sauce (or to taste). Stir to combine. Garnish with green onion, cilantro, and more hot sauce.

PER SERVING

Calories	339
Fat	12.8g
Carbs	35.5g
Fiber	4.7g
Sugars	10.4g
Protein	24.7g
WW Points	9

SERVES 2

Asian hot sauce (e.g., Sriracha; optional)

1 tbsp minced jalapeño

¼ c finely diced red onion

1½ tbsp minced fresh ginger

2 tbsp low-sodium soy sauce or gluten-free tamari, divided

2 tbsp rice vinegar, divided

2 garlic cloves, minced

6 tbsp pineapple juice, divided

8 oz tempeh, cubed

1 tbsp cornstarch mixed into 2 tbsp water

4 c (10 oz) shredded cabbage

green onions, sliced (optional)

cilantro (optional)

pineapple stir-fry

Quick, easy, and delicious. This light stir-fry doesn't feel like a slimmed-down dish. It's still big on taste without coconut milk. If you'd like to add another vegetable to bulk up the dish, try broccoli. Serve over brown rice or quinoa.

PER SERVING
(WITHOUT RICE)

Calories	215
Fat	5.7g
Carbs	30.7g
Fiber	4.6g
Sugars	18.2g
Protein	12.8g
WW Points	6

SERVES 2

- ½ c vegetable broth, divided
- 4 green onions, sliced
- 3 garlic cloves, minced
- 1 tbsp minced fresh ginger root
- pinch red pepper flakes
- 1 tbsp brown rice vinegar
- 1 tbsp low-sodium soy sauce or gluten-free tamari
- 1 tbsp sweet red chili sauce
- 1 red bell pepper, seeded and sliced into strips
- 1 c pineapple chunks
- ¼ c pineapple juice
- 1 c diced tofu
- 1 tsp cornstarch mixed into 2 tbsp water
- cilantro (optional)
- Asian hot sauce (e.g., Sriracha; optional)

Line skillet with a thin layer of broth. Sauté white and light green parts of the onions (reserving dark parts for later), garlic, ginger, and a dash or two red pepper flakes for a few minutes, until fragrant. Add vinegar, soy sauce or tamari, sweet red chili sauce, red bell pepper, and a splash of broth—enough so there is a thin layer of liquid in the skillet. Continue to sauté, adding broth as necessary, until peppers are tender but still crisp. Add pineapple chunks, juice, and tofu, and stir to combine. Add cornstarch and continue to cook and stir, until sauce has thickened. Stir in 2–3 tbsp cilantro, if desired. Then garnish with leftover green onion and additional cilantro as desired. Add a drizzle of hot sauce for a spicy dish, if desired, and serve.

Chef's Note Rice vinegar may be substituted for the brown rice vinegar.

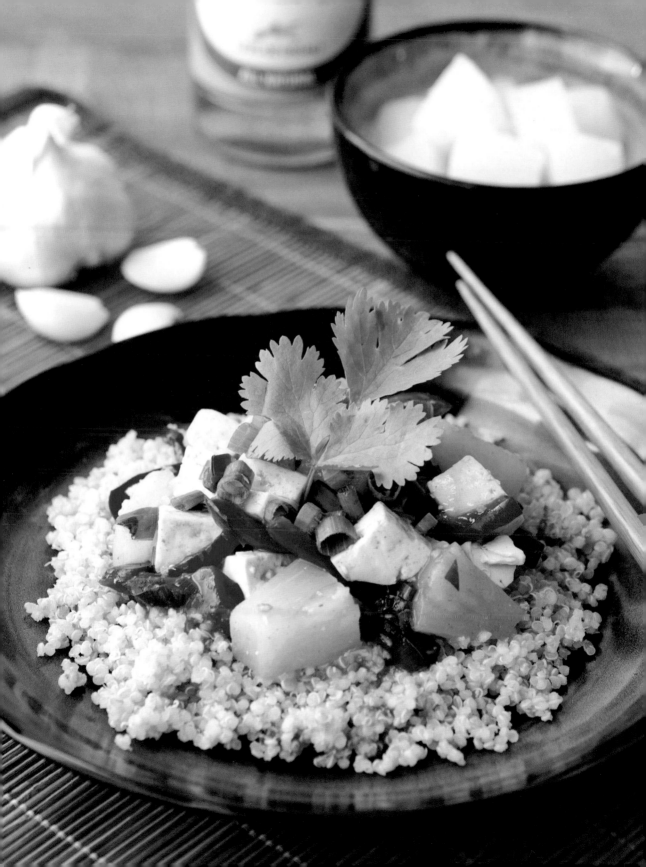

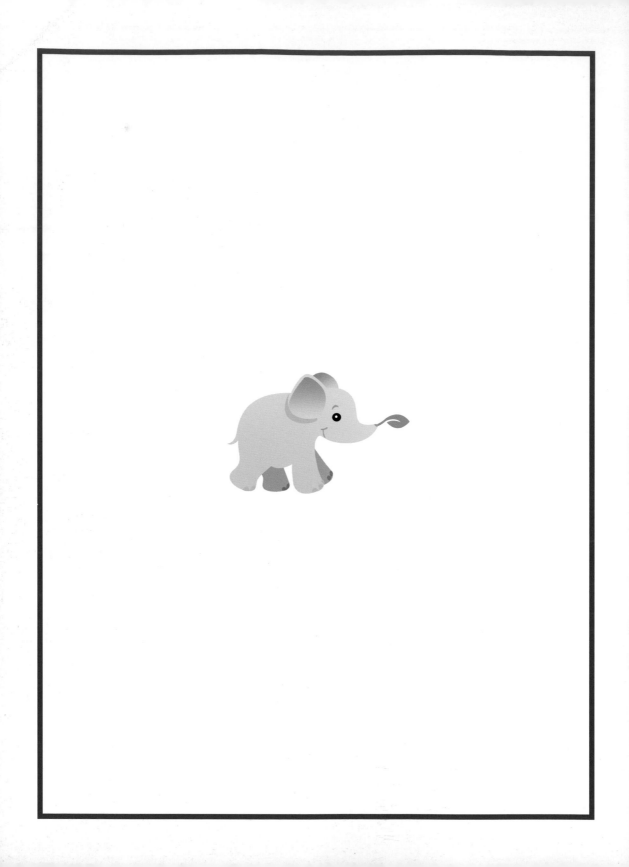

satisfying sides

smoky apple baked beans

PER SERVING
(ABOUT ½ CUP)

Calories	169
Fat	0.7g
Carbs	33.8g
Fiber	9.1g
Sugars	10.7g
Protein	8.4g
WW Points	4

SERVES 6

- vegetable broth
- 1 small onion, diced
- 4–6 garlic cloves, minced
- ¼ c tomato sauce
- 2 tbsp molasses
- 2–3 tbsp pure maple syrup
- 1 tbsp Dijon mustard
- ½ c unsweetened applesauce, divided
- few drops liquid smoke
- 1–2 tsp chili powder
- 1 15-oz can white beans, drained and rinsed
- 1 15-oz can kidney beans, drained and rinsed
- 2 tbsp barbecue sauce (optional)
- cayenne or hot sauce to taste
- smoked paprika

I love (and my parents are addicted to) the Baked Beans recipe in *The Happy Herbivore Cookbook*. I wanted to re-vamp that recipe slightly—add in some apple for a natural sweetness and incorporate a smoky element. Win! I love these beans and, after a trip to Ireland, have also taken a liking to eating them at breakfast with toast or oven-roasted potatoes. Try it!

Line a large pot with a thin layer of vegetable broth and sauté onion and garlic over high heat until onion is translucent and most of the broth has evaporated. Stir in tomato sauce, molasses, 2 tbsp maple syrup, Dijon, ¼ cup applesauce, plus a few drops of liquid smoke (a little goes a long way). Then add 1–2 tsp chili powder and beans. Stir well, cover, and bring to a boil, then immediately reduce heat to low. Simmer 10–20 minutes until warm and white beans have taken on a brown coloring. Add remaining ¼ cup applesauce and barbecue sauce if using, and stir to combine. Taste, adding additional maple syrup, chili powder, cayenne/hot sauce, or liquid smoke as de-sired. Add a few dashes of smoked paprika and serve slightly warm.

Chef's Note Any white beans, such as navy, cannellini, or butter bean, will work in this recipe.

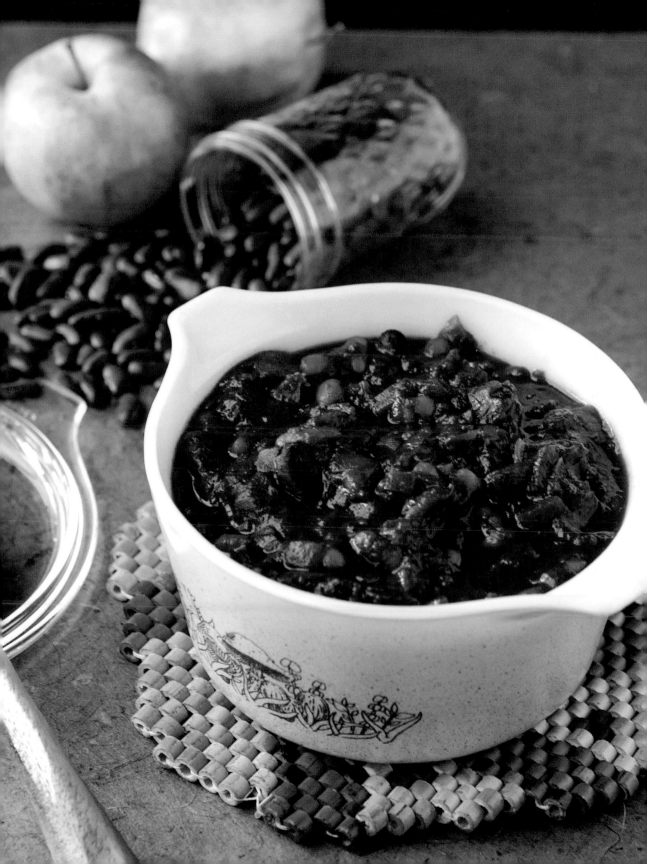

PER SERVING

Calories 129
Fat. 0.4g
Carbs 28.1g
Fiber 4.7g
Sugars. 9.6g
Protein 3.8g
WW Points 3

SERVES 2

3 c cubed sweet
potato

1–2 tbsp vegan mayo or
plain vegan yogurt

chipotle powder

2 green onions, sliced

smoked paprika
(garnish) (optional)

Chef's Note I find this salad is
even more flavorful after it's
rested overnight in the fridge.

chipotle sweet potato salad

Sweet potatoes are a hidden surprise in this fiery potato salad. If you'd like to make a meal out of the salad, try adding in some black beans and a little avocado, plus a dash of ground cumin for kicks.

Bring a large pot of water to a boil, add sweet potato, and boil until just fork-tender. Drain, rinse with cold water, and then chill overnight or for several hours—until cold. Once potatoes are cool, add mayo and stir to coat. Add a light dash of chipotle (a little goes a long way!) and stir to coat. Taste, adding more chipotle as desired, plus salt and pepper if desired. Add green onions and stir again. Garnish with a few green onion slices and smoked paprika if desired.

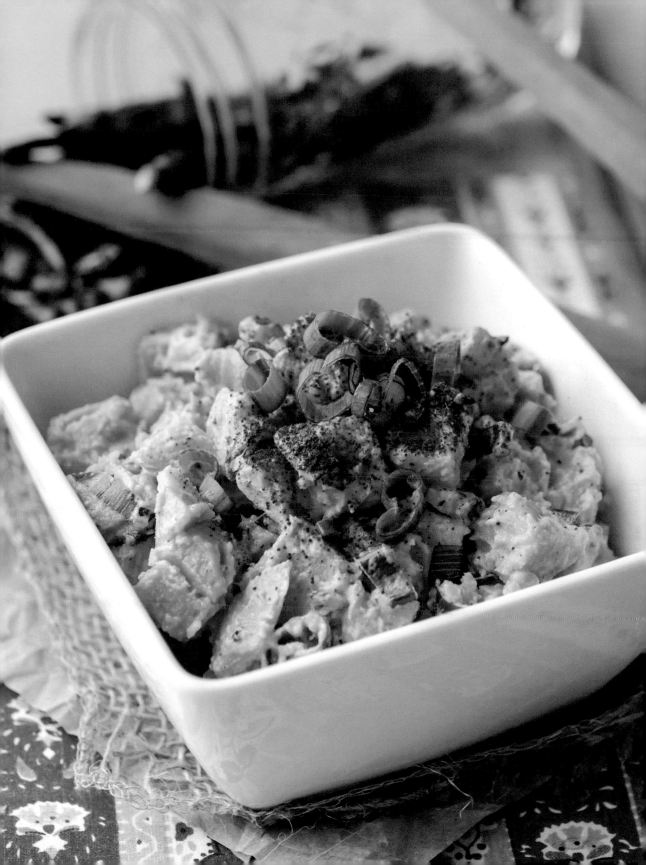

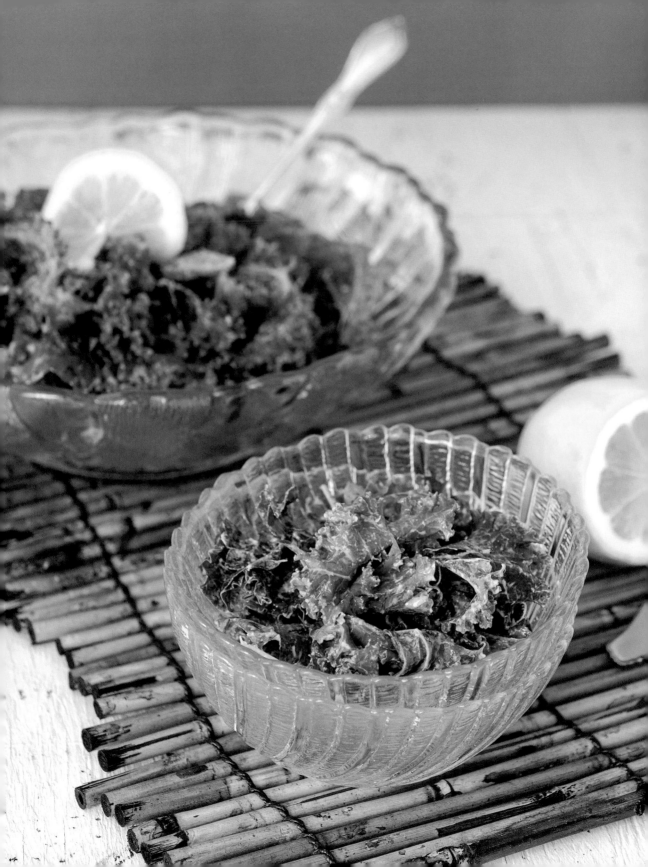

kale slaw

I'm always looking for more ways to eat raw kale and this slaw makes it easy on me. It has the creamy taste of a traditional side slaw, but it's made with vegan yogurt instead of mayonnaise for a healthier twist.

Place kale in a mixing bowl and then massage it, like you're crumbling dough in your hands. Keep massaging until the kale softens a little, reduces in volume, and becomes a little brighter in color. Then use your hands to mix kale with yogurt until well covered. Add Dijon and mix again. Taste, adding more Dijon as desired. For a fun variation, try adding a touch of lemon juice for a lemony kale slaw.

PER SERVING

Calories	147
Fat	2.2g
Carbs	28g
Fiber	5.4g
Sugars	1.1g
Protein	9.8g
WW Points	4

SERVES 2

- 8 c chopped kale
- 2–3 tbsp plain vegan yogurt
- 1–2 tsp Dijon mustard
- lemon juice (optional)

I find rounding out a meal with a side or two always makes it feel more satisfying and exciting. Baby carrots, apple slices, cucumber slices, celery, baked potato, sweet potato, grapes, jicama sticks—these are easy (and healthy) additions to a plate.

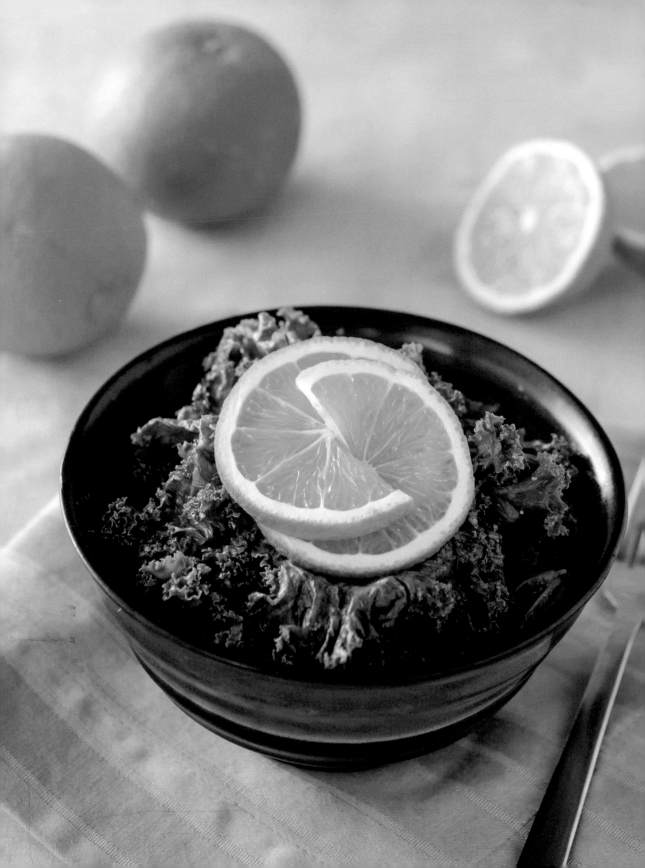

asian orange kale salad

The delicious orange-flavored sauce in this recipe can make you love anything, even raw kale. Incidentally, my brain is always tripping with this recipe and I end up saying "Agent Orange" Kale Salad instead. Oy vey.

Place kale in a large bowl then massage it, like you're crumbling dough in your hands. Keep massaging until the kale softens a little, reduces in volume, and becomes a little brighter in color. A little bit of salt can really help with this. Set massaged kale aside and prepare dressing by whisking remaining ingredients together. Pour over kale, stirring to combine well. Serve immediately.

Chef's Notes

» If you want a cool salad, make dressing first and store it in the fridge or freezer while massaging the kale.

» Rice vinegar may be substituted for the brown rice vinegar

» My friend Jennifer passed this kale salad tip along to me: "I soak my kale in hot water to soften it up for salads. I find this method also helps make the dressing 'stick' to the kale a bit better."

PER SERVING

Calories	209
Fat	2.1g
Carbs	43.7g
Fiber	4.8g
Sugars	18.6g
Protein	8.3g
WW Points	6

SERVES 2

- 6 c chopped kale
- 2 tbsp orange marmalade or jam
- 1 tbsp yellow miso
- 1 tsp sweet red chili sauce
- 1 tbsp brown rice vinegar
- 1 tsp low-sodium soy sauce or gluten-free tamari
- 1 tbsp vegetable broth
- 1 tsp orange zest
  juice of 2 orange slices, about 2–3 tbsp

PER SERVING
CREAMY KALE SALAD /
SWEET KALE SALAD

Calories	142/118
Fat	3.9g/1g
Carbs	23.6g/25.2g
Fiber	6.2g/4.6g
Sugars	3.4g/3.7g
Protein	7.5g/5.6g
WW Points	4/3

creamy kale salad

The idea of massaging kale with hummus came to me by way of the Esselstyn clan. (I love that family!) Massaging raw kale with hummus makes it softer, plus the hummus lends itself to be a fuss-free creamy dressing with a protein boost. I love this satisfying salad!

SERVES 2

- 4 c (about ½ bunch) kale, de-stemmed and torn into bite-size pieces
- 4–6 tbsp plain or red pepper hummus
- ¼ c red onion, diced
- chickpeas (optional)
- ½ c cherry tomatoes, sliced or 1 red bell pepper, seeded and diced
- 1 lemon

Place kale in a bowl with ¼ cup (4 tbsp) hummus and use your hands to rub together, massaging kale until kale is softer, breaks down in volume, and is well coated with hummus. Add more hummus, 1 tbsp at a time, if needed or desired. Stir in onion, chickpeas, and cherry tomatoes or bell pepper. Add juice of ½ lemon (or ¼ if it's very big) and mix. Taste, adding more lemon if desired.

sweet kale salad

A reminder that simple is ridiculously awesome.

SERVES 2

- 1 large sweet potato
- 4 c (about ½ bunch) kale, de-stemmed and torn into bite-size pieces

Cook sweet potato and when cool, pull away skin. In a large bowl, combine with kale and, using your hands, rub together, massaging until the kale is softer and well coated.

Chef's Note Add a few dashes of garam masala for a twist!

parmesan greens

I love kale and this is one of my favorite ways to eat it. A hint of lemon, a touch of heat, and a sprinkling of Parmesan—what's not to love? These greens are a nice addition to any meal.

Remove kale from stems and tear into bite-sized pieces; set aside. Line a skillet with a thin layer of broth. Add garlic and a dash of red pepper flakes and sauté over high heat until garlic is golden, fragrant, and the broth has cooked off. Add enough broth so there is a thin layer coating the bottom of the skillet and add kale. Continue to cook over high, stirring kale constantly until it softens and turns brighter in color, about 1–2 minutes. Make sure the minced garlic is coating the kale as you stir. Turn off heat and stir well. Add a pinch of lemon zest and several dashes of vegan Parmesan cheese, as desired, stir again, and serve.

PER SERVING

Calories	156
Fat	2.7g
Carbs	29.6g
Fiber	5.7g
Sugars	0g
Protein	10.2g
WW Points	4

SERVES 2

1 bunch kale
   vegetable broth
3–5 garlic cloves, minced
   red pepper flakes
   zest of small lemon
   AJ's Vegan Parmesan
   (pg. 271)

Chef's Note You can use broccoli in place of the kale in this recipe. Steam broccoli until fork-tender, then toss cooked garlic and chili with broccoli. Add lemon zest and vegan Parmesan before serving.

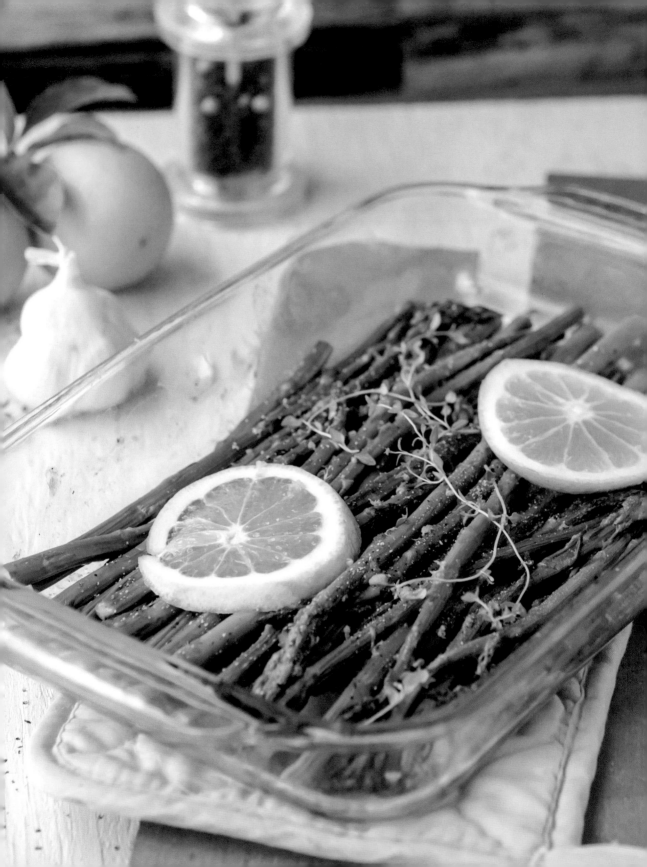

lemony asparagus

The glaze in this recipe is so delicious it shouldn't be limited to just asparagus but my, my, how it makes asparagus shine! I also like this sauce over green beans, and some of my testers took to tossing it with potatoes and chickpeas, too.

Steam or oven-roast asparagus at 425°F for 15 minutes. Meanwhile, combine all other ingredients in a saucepan, whisking to combine. Bring to a boil then reduce heat to low, and simmer, stirring constantly, until it thickens like a glaze. Taste, adding more Dijon or lemon juice as desired. Toss with asparagus and garnish with lemon slices and a little zest, adding cracked fresh black pepper and salt if desired.

PER SERVING

Calories	38
Fat	0.3g
Carbs	8.2g
Fiber	2.4g
Sugars	2.6g
Protein	2.3g
WW Points	1

SERVES 2

- 1 bunch asparagus, trimmed
- ½ c low-sodium vegetable broth
- 1–2 tsp Dijon mustard
- 4–6 thyme springs, de-stemmed
  dash onion powder
  dash garlic powder
- 1 tsp cornstarch
- ½ –1 tsp lemon juice (fresh is best)

citrus couscous

PER SERVING
[¾ CUP]

Calories 185
Fat. 0.4g
Carbs 40.7g
Fiber 4.8g
Sugars. 12.3g
Protein 5.5g
WW Points 5

I like to eat couscous for breakfast topped with a little plain or vanilla vegan yogurt, or as a side salad with sliced green onion mixed in. It's also one of my favorite fall and winter dishes when oranges and grapefruit are at their peaks.

SERVES 2

½ c water

6 tbsp uncooked whole-wheat couscous

1 orange

1 grapefruit (I use pink grapefruit)

2 tbsp or more minced fresh mint

orange zest (optional)

Bring water to a boil, combine with couscous, and stir. It won't look like it's enough water, but it absorbs well. Fluff with a spoon and set aside. Peel orange and then slice each wedge in half. Cut grapefruit in half, squeezing juice from one half into couscous, really using your fingers to get all the juice out. Peel the other grapefruit half, then slice each wedge in half and stir into couscous with orange slices. Add 2 tbsp minced fresh mint; stir to combine. Taste, adding more mint if desired. For a stronger citrus flavor or scent, try adding a little orange zest, but don't add too much or it'll taste bitter.

Chef's Note For a gluten-free option, use cooked quinoa (1⅓ cups or thereabouts) in place of the couscous.

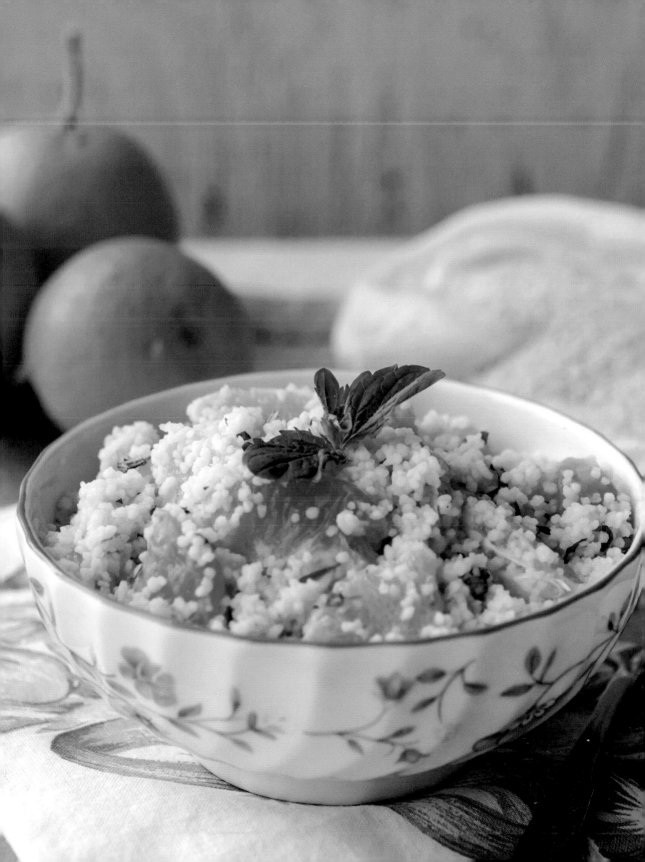

PER SERVING
(ABOUT ⅓ CUP)

Calories 51
Fat. 0.1g
Carbs 10.6g
Fiber 0.8g
Sugars. 0g
Protein 1.8g
WW Points. 1

SERVES 5

½ c water

6 tbsp uncooked whole-wheat couscous

1–2 small lemons (zest and juice)

3 tbsp minced fresh basil

1–2 tbsp vegan mayo or plain vegan yogurt

Chef's Note For a gluten-free option, use cooked quinoa (1⅓ cups or thereabouts) in place of the couscous.

lemony couscous

"So nice they named it twice." Couscous is a grain, and traditionally a meat or vegetable stew is served over couscous (and simply referred to as "couscous"). Here I'm letting couscous shine front and center in a light but filling lemon side dish. To make a meal or larger salad, add sliced green onion or red onion, cherry tomatoes, and chickpeas or white beans.

Bring water to a boil, combine with couscous, and stir. It won't look like it's enough water, but it absorbs well. Fluff with a spoon and set aside. Add 1 tsp lemon zest and juice of half a lemon. Stir to combine and taste, adding more lemon juice if desired. Stir in 3 tbsp minced fresh basil and mayo or yogurt. Add salt and pepper, then taste, adding more lemon juice, zest, or basil.

✔ SOY-FREE   ✔ GLUTEN-FREE   ✔ QUICK   ✔ BUDGET   ✔ PANTRY

easy mashed potatoes & gravy

I know, everyone knows how to make mashed potatoes: You mash a potato! So this isn't even a recipe, really, as much as a suggestion of how to make flavorful mashed potatoes without milk and butter to accompany some of the meals in this book. I'm also including my Quick Gravy recipe (pg. 188).

Cube 1–2 large baking potatoes (skins optional) and boil until fork-tender. Drain and beat with an electric beater. Add 1–2 tbsp garlic powder and ½–1 tbsp onion powder or onion flakes, plus a splash of plain nondairy milk, and beat again, adding more liquid as necessary to achieve the right consistency. Taste, adding more spices as desired, plus salt and pepper to taste.

Alternatively, forgo the spices and add a squirt or two of Dijon mustard (all Dijon mustards vary in strength, so this is very much a "to-taste" method).

PER SERVING

Calories 147
Fat. 1.2g
Carbs 30.8g
Fiber 4.4g
Sugars. 1.5g
Protein 4.2g
WW Points 4

SERVES 2

2 baking potatoes
1–2 tbsp garlic powder (optional)
½ –1 tbsp onion powder or onion flakes (optional)
nondairy milk
Dijon mustard (optional)

PER SERVING
QUICK GRAVY (ABOUT ½ CUP) /
OVEN FRIES

Calories 73/131
Fat. 0.7g/0.1g
Carbs 12.8g/29.7g
Fiber 3.4g/3.7g
Sugars. 1.1g/1.3g
Protein 5.9g/3.4g
WW Points 2/3

SERVES 4

¼ c nutritional yeast

¼ c white whole-wheat
flour

2 c low-sodium
vegetable broth

1–2 tbsp low-sodium soy
sauce or gluten-free
tamari

1 tsp onion powder

¼ tsp garlic powder

SINGLE SERVING

1 potato

quick gravy

In a small nonstick skillet, whisk nutritional yeast and flour together and toast over medium heat until it smells toasty, about 4 minutes. Transfer to a medium saucepan and whisk in remaining ingredients. Bring to a boil and allow to thicken as desired. Add salt and pepper to taste. For an even thicker gravy, mix 1 tbsp of cornstarch with 2 tbsp of water and pour it into the gravy.

Chef's Note For a gluten-free gravy, use brown rice flour.

oven fries

Because you can't have a bean burger without fries!

Preheat oven to 425°F. Line cookie sheet with parchment paper and set aside. Cut potato into fry-size strips about the size of your pinkie finger. It's important they are as even in size as possible. Bake 10 minutes, flipping the fries after 7 minutes have passed. Then switch to broil (high) for another minute or two until the fries are golden—but be careful; they can burn fast.

everyday mushroom gravy

You might remember this gravy recipe from *Everyday Happy Herbivore*. It's so great, versatile, and low calorie that I had to include it again!

In a skillet, whisk water with soy sauce or tamari, 1 tbsp of nutritional yeast, onion powder, garlic powder, and ground ginger. Bring to a boil and add mushrooms, sprinkling them generously with Italian seasoning (a good 10 shakes). Continue to sauté over medium-high heat until the mushrooms are brown and soft, about 3 minutes. Meanwhile whisk nondairy milk with cornstarch and remaining 1 tbsp of nutritional yeast. Add a very light dash of ground nutmeg, if desired. Pour over mushrooms, stirring to combine. Reduce heat to low and continue to cook until thick and gravylike, about 5 minutes. Add black pepper to taste (I like it really peppery) and a few more shakes of Italian seasoning unless you were very generous before. Taste again, adding a pinch of salt if necessary. Set aside for a few minutes before serving to let the flavors merge.

PER SERVING
(ABOUT ¼ CUP)

Calories 60
Fat. 1.4g
Carbs 8.9g
Sugars. 1.2g
Fiber 1.4g
Protein 5.6g
WW Points 2

MAKES 1 CUP

- 1 c water
- 2 tbsp low-sodium soy sauce or gluten-free tamari
- 2 tbsp nutritional yeast, divided
- ¼ tsp granulated onion powder
- ¼ tsp granulated garlic powder
- ¼ tsp ground ginger
- 8 oz white or brown mushrooms, sliced
- Italian seasoning
- ½ c nondairy milk
- 2 tbsp cornstarch
- dash of ground nutmeg (optional)

Chef's Note For a smoky-flavored gravy, substitute smoked paprika for the ground nutmeg, and add more to taste.

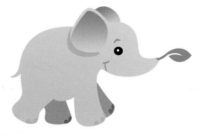

dips, snacks & appetizers

zucchini "mozzarella" sticks

PER SERVING
(1 STICK, WITHOUT MARINARA)

Calories	21
Fat	0.3g
Carbs	3.6g
Fiber	0.7g
Sugars	0.5g
Protein	1.2g
WW Points	1

MAKES 24

- 2 zucchini
- ¾ c whole-wheat bread crumbs
- 3 tbsp AJ's Vegan Parmesan (pg. 271)
- ½ tsp garlic powder
- ⅓ c nondairy milk
- pizza sauce or Marinara Sauce (pg. 263), warmed

Chef's Note You can make your own bread crumbs by toasting a piece of bread and then chopping it up into crumbs in your blender or food processor.

I wasn't much of a cheese eater when I was a vegetarian, but I loved mozzarella sticks. Actually, I think I just liked the marinara sauce, because I could leave the actual mozzarella sticks. But the sauce? Now we're talking. Here's how I scratch the itch now: all the dipping into marinara sauce I want, plus I'm getting in a serving of vegetables!

Preheat oven to 400°F. Line a cookie sheet with parchment paper and set aside. Cut zucchini into sticks ½-inch thick and set aside. If bread crumbs are coarse, grind to a fine consistency using a mortar and pestle or food processor. Mix crumbs with vegan Parmesan and garlic, plus a few dashes of salt and pepper. Place crumb mixture into a shallow bowl. Pour nondairy milk into another shallow bowl. Dip zucchini into the nondairy milk and then press all sides into the crumb mixture. Transfer coated zucchini sticks to cookie sheet. Bake 15–20 minutes, until the breading is golden and zucchini tender. Serve with warm marinara sauce for dipping.

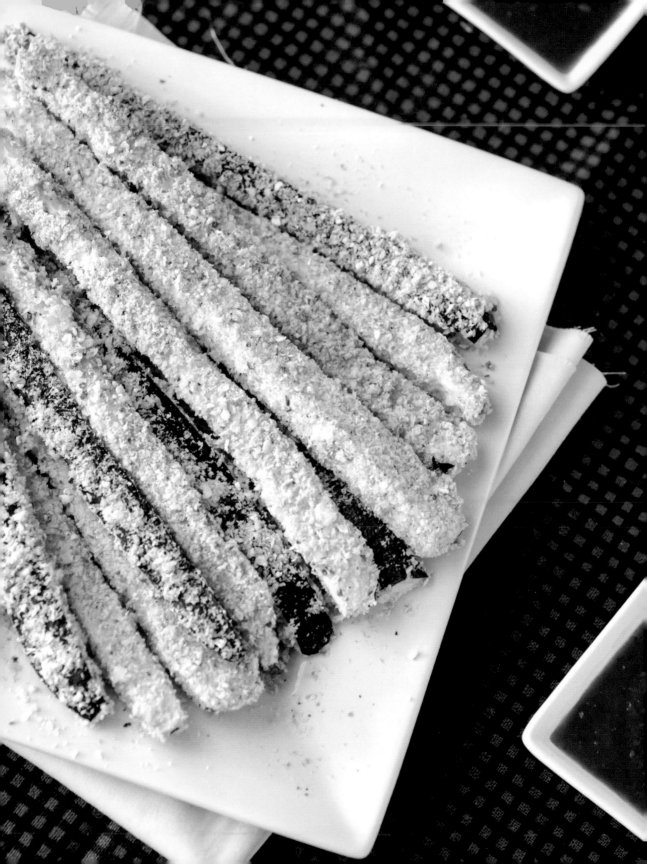

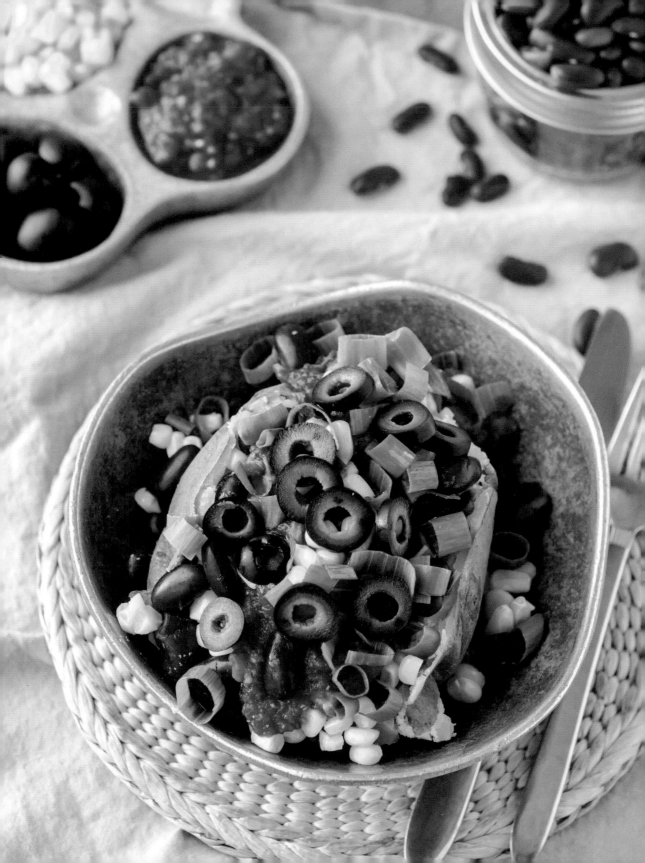

loaded mexican potato

Sometimes when I get a hankering for nachos or chips and salsa, I make one of these healthy potatoes for a twist instead. I get all the taste satisfaction but for a fraction of the calories. The secret is the potato. It's big and filling but has fewer calories than baked corn chips. If you miss the crunch, try crumbling a few corn chips over top. You can also add black or kidney beans for a boost of protein.

Bake, boil, steam, slow-cook (Slow-Cooked Baked Potatoes, pg. 268), or microwave potato. Slice in half and top with remaining ingredients.

PER SERVING

Calories	223
Fat	2.6g
Carbs	47.3g
Fiber	7.8g
Sugars	6.9g
Protein	7.1g
WW Points	6

SINGLE SERVING

- 1 potato
- ½ c salsa
- ¼ c corn
- 2 tbsp sliced black olives
- 1 green onion, sliced
- ½ c cooked black or kidney beans (optional)
- broken corn chips (optional)
- Quick Nacho Sauce (pg. 212)
- guacamole or pea guacamole (optional)

Chef's Note You can make healthier corn chips by cutting corn tortillas into triangles and crisping in the oven or toaster oven for a few minutes at 350°F.

PER SERVING
(BASE INGREDIENTS ONLY)

Calories 338
Fat. 2.6g
Carbs 73g
Fiber 11.8g
Sugars. 6.3g
Protein 14.2g
WW Points 9

SINGLE SERVING

- 1 potato
- 1 c vegetarian chili or black bean soup
- 2 green onions, sliced
- 1 tomato, diced
- 2 tbsp corn (thawed, if using frozen)
- Vegan Sour Cream (pg. 262) (optional)
- guacamole or low-fat guacamole (optional)
- Tempeh Bacon (pg. 36) (optional)
- hot sauce

game day loaded potato

This is similar to my Loaded Mexican Potato but with Super Bowl Sunday and "potato skins" in mind. These spuds also scratch the itch when you want chili and cheese fries! On a funny note, my friend Kim tested this recipe out on her family for me, and wrote back, "Kids want it on a weekly basis during football season. (They said it will make having to watch football more tolerable. LOL.)" Ha!

Steam, bake, boil, slow-cook (Slow-Cooked Baked Potatoes, pg. 268), or microwave potato. Place in a wide bowl or on a plate, then slice in half long-ways, mashing the middle. Top with chili or soup, onions, tomato, corn, sour cream, guacamole, and bacon if using. Drizzle generously with hot sauce.

Chef's Note You can use homemade or canned vegetarian chili or black bean soup. I typically use leftovers to make these potatoes for lunch the day after having soup or chili from dinner. For chili ideas, see the Soups, Stews & Savory Pies section (pg. 103). For black bean soup, check out my Cuban Black Bean Soup recipe in *Happy Herbivore Abroad*.

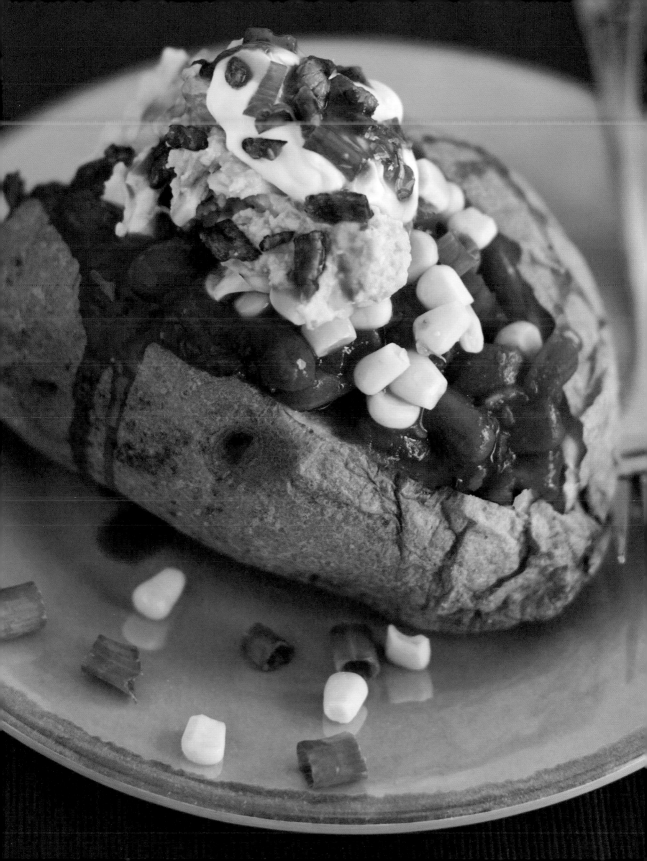

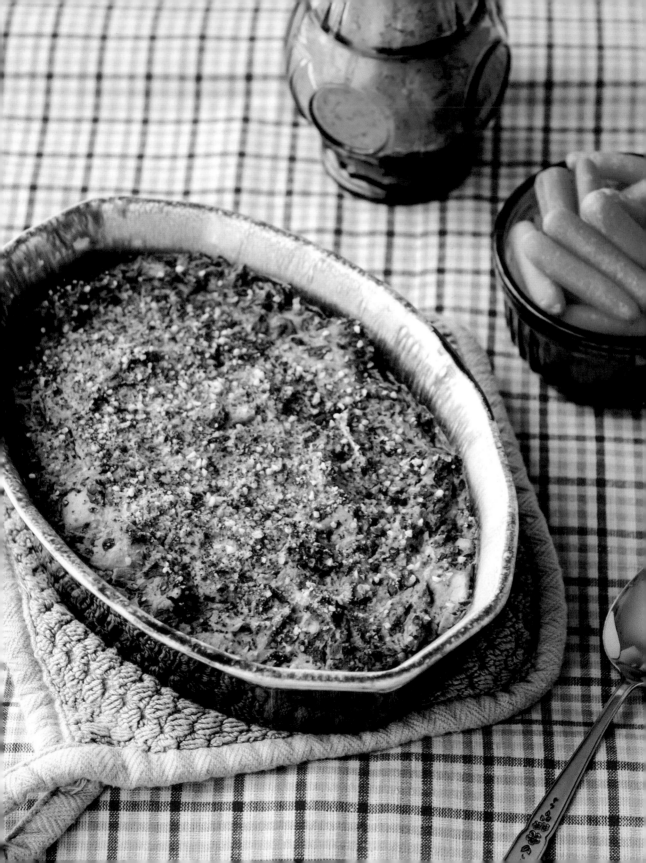

spinach & artichoke dip

Spinach and artichoke dip that's good for you? Possible! Spread this dip on crusty whole grain bread or serve with crackers, raw vegetables, and/or whole-wheat pita warmed and cut into triangles. It's addictive!

Preheat oven to 350°F. Grab an 8-inch glass pie or casserole dish and set aside. Cook spinach according to package instructions, taking care to press out all the excess water and set aside. In a small pot or skillet, sauté garlic and onion with ¼ cup vegetable broth over high heat until garlic is golden, onion is translucent, and most of the liquid has evaporated. Transfer onion-garlic mixture to a food processor or blender with beans and nondairy milk. Whiz until smooth and creamy. Add nutritional yeast and Dijon (use less if your brand is spicy or strong), plus salt and pepper, if desired, and blend again. If your artichoke hearts are big, quarter or chop them. Transfer spinach, bean mixture, and artichoke hearts to pot from earlier, mixing to combine. Pour into baking dish and spread out in an even layer. Bake for 10–20 minutes or until warm and the top is golden. Generously garnish with vegan Parmesan and a few light dashes of smoked paprika (if using).

PER SERVING

Calories 195
Fat. 2g
Carbs 30.2g
Fiber 12.9g
Sugars. 1.2g
Protein 17g
WW Points 4

SERVES 4

12 oz frozen spinach
4–8 garlic cloves, minced
1 small onion, diced
¼ c vegetable broth or spinach water
1 c cooked white beans
½ c nondairy milk
½ c nutritional yeast
1–2 tsp Dijon mustard
1 14-oz can artichoke hearts (in water, not oil), drained
AJ's Vegan Parmesan (pg. 271) (optional)
smoked paprika (optional garnish)

Chef's Notes

» This dip is for garlic lovers: Add as much garlic as you like. If you don't love garlic, you can scale it back, but I recommend at least 2 good-size cloves.

» Any white beans, such as navy, cannellini, or butter bean, will work in this recipe.

"cheese" ball

MAKES 1 BALL

- ½ c cooked chickpeas
- ⅓ block of extra-firm tofu (about 5 oz)
- 5 tbsp nutritional yeast
- 1 tbsp yellow miso
- few drops liquid smoke
- few drops agave nectar
- 1 tsp yellow mustard
- ½ tsp onion powder
- ½ tsp garlic powder

I was never much of a cheese fanatic, but oh how I loved cheese balls at Christmas. A friend of mine turned me on to a vegan recipe for a "cheese" ball, and it was good, but contained way too many nuts for my liking so I set out to develop a low-fat version. I love this "cheese" ball and make it any time I'm having company over or going to a party. It never lasts more than a few minutes!

Combine all ingredients in a good processor until smooth and pastelike. Spoon out into a metal bowl, then use a rubber spatula to scrape and smooth it into a ball. Cover with plastic wrap and chill for a few hours. Transfer to your serving plate and garnish with smoked paprika and almond slices on the outside, if desired.

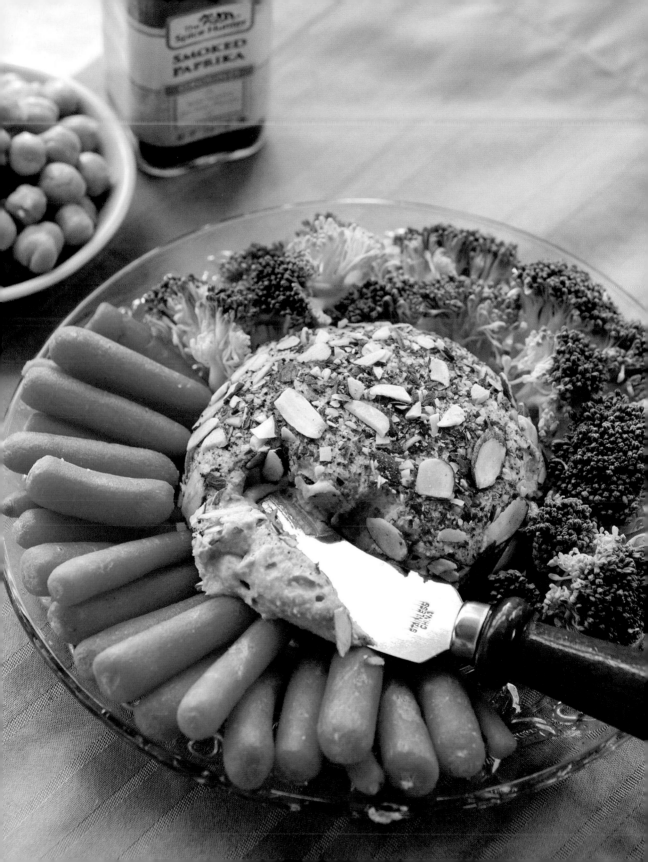

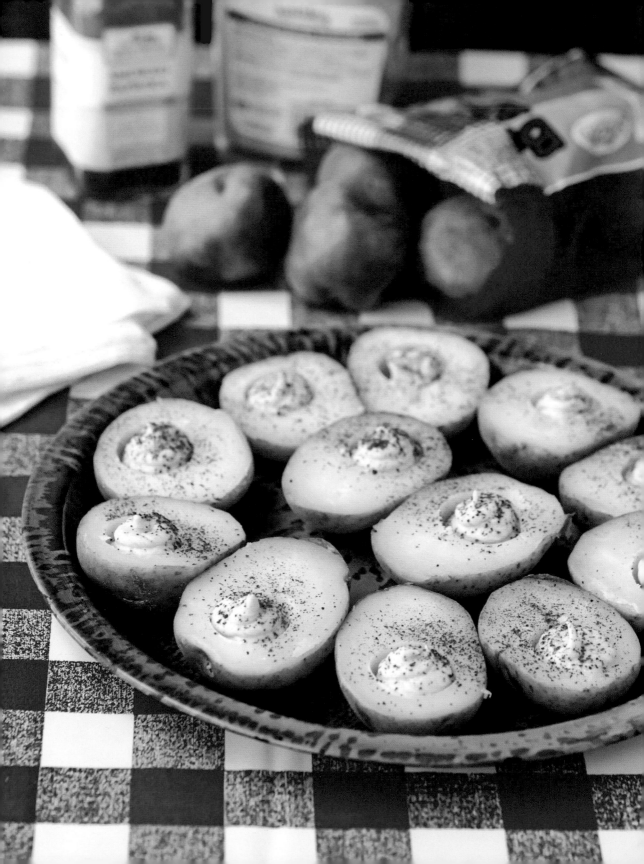

deviled "eggs"

Ann Esselstyn taught me how to make these incredible faux deviled eggs. Her recipe was simple: hummus, Dijon mustard, green onions, and paprika. I added a little black salt to give the deviled eggs a little more egg flavor and added some additional seasonings my mother used in her deviled eggs recipe as well. I swear I could eat two dozen of these eggs all by myself!

Boil potatoes until fork-tender, then let cool completely. Meanwhile, mix hummus, Dijon, garlic powder, and onion powder together, plus a pinch of black salt, stirring to combine. (Add hot sauce here if you prefer a spicy deviled egg.) Taste, adding more Dijon or black salt to taste, then set aside. Once potatoes cool, slice in half long-ways and use a little spoon or melon baller to scoop out a small circle of the potato flesh (this is your "egg"). Spoon hummus mixture into the hole and garnish with paprika.

PER EGG

Calories	69
Fat	0.6g
Carbs	14.4g
Fiber	18g
Sugars	0.9g
Protein	2.1g
WW Points	0

MAKES 12

- 6 small red potatoes
- ¼ c hummus (plain)
- 1 tsp Dijon mustard
- ¼ tsp garlic powder
- ¼ tsp onion powder
- pinch black salt
- hot sauce (optional)
- paprika or smoked paprika (garnish)

Chef's Note Black salt is also called *kala namak*. Not to be confused with Hawaiian black lava salt.

tempeh wings

MAKES 16

1 8-oz pkg tempeh
3–4 tbsp hot sauce
¼ c plain vegan yogurt

Chef's Note For a soy-free option, try tossing the sauce with oven-roasted cauliflower florets. A few restaurants in LA make "wings" with battered cauliflower and wing sauce.

My healthy answer to hot wings. I'm always getting requests for wings or wing sauce recipes and this is my easy (and healthy) solution.

Preheat oven to 375°F. Line a cookie sheet with parchment paper. Slice tempeh short-ways into strips, yielding roughly 16 strips. Bake for 10–15 minutes, or until slightly crisp, flipping the wings at the halfway point if you can. If your tempeh strips are being stubborn, try broiling them for a minute or two—but keep a watchful eye so they don't burn. Meanwhile, whisk 3 tbsp hot sauce with yogurt until well combined. Taste, adding more hot sauce for a hotter sauce. When the tempeh is done, coat with the sauce or dip!

sweet potato chips

No fancy dehydrator required—just an oven! When my friend Dirk made these, he said, "Nothing but good, cheap, easy, available ingredients, and earthy goodness done just right." Couldn't have said it better myself!

Preheat oven to 375°F and line a cookie sheet with parchment paper. Slice sweet potato thinly, about ⅛-inch thick (I recommend using a mandolin or veggie slicer for uniform precision). Place chips on parchment paper and bake for 5 minutes. Flip over and bake another 3 minutes. Check and bake up to 5 more minutes until the sides are curly and lifting—but be careful not to burn. (Baking time depends on chip thickness, so it can vary.) If your chips are being stubborn, try broiling for 30 seconds or so for added crispness, but be careful not to burn. Allow chips to cool; they crisp slightly as they cool.

PER SERVING
(ABOUT 15 CHIPS)

Calories	51
Fat	0.1g
Carbs	11.8g
Fiber	1.9g
Sugars	3.7g
Protein	1.1g
WW Points	1

SERVES 2

1 sweet potato

kale chips

A crunchy, healthy snack full of super green goodness! This is my method for baking these delicious chips—no oil added and no dehydrator required!

PER SERVING
(ABOUT ¼ OF THE CHIPS)

Calories 67
Fat. 0.9g
Carbs 13.4g
Fiber 2.7g
Sugars. 0g
Protein 4.4g
WW Points 2

SERVES 4

1 bunch kale, de-stemmed

spices

Preheat oven (toaster oven works best) to 225°F. Tear kale into pieces (uniformity is more important than size—but they shrink down so don't make the pieces too small). Place kale on a nonstick cookie sheet or a cookie sheet lined with parchment paper. Sprinkle generously with spices such as sea salt, nutritional yeast, Old Bay Seasoning (my favorite), ground ginger, garlic salt, or anything you like. Bake for 7–10 minutes until dark green and crispy, but be careful not to burn!

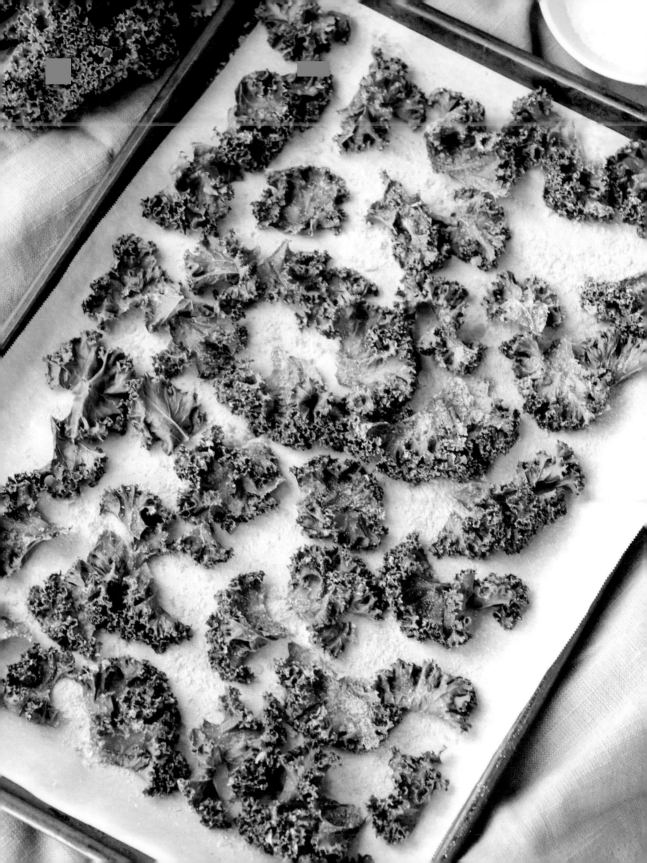

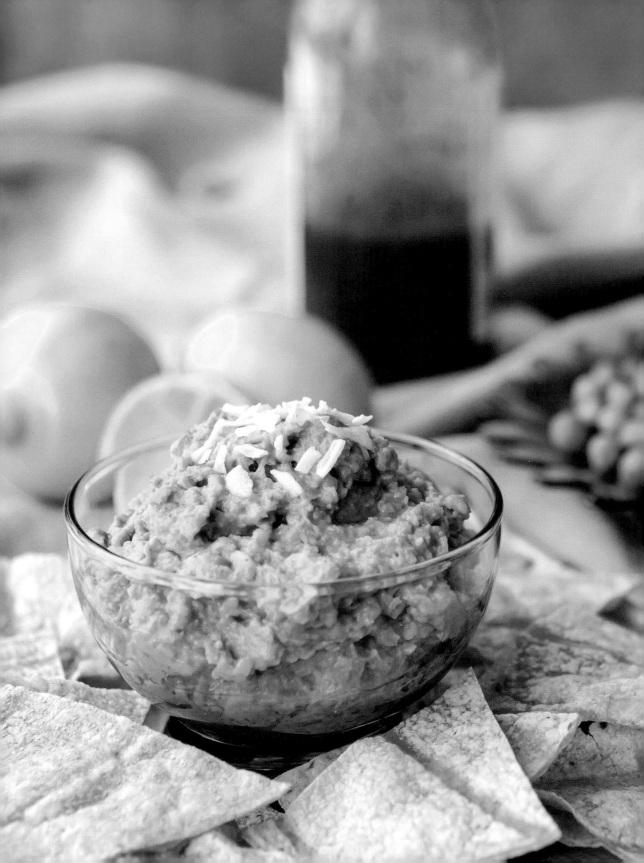

sweet pea guacamole

Peas are the not-so-secret secret ingredient in this recipe. Peas help cut the fat of traditional guacamole while adding in an extra boost of protein and a hint of sweetness. I always serve this at summer parties and it's usually the first thing to go! As a side note, after my friend Kim made this guac for her girls, the next morning a note appeared on the fridge: "Mas pea guac, por favor." That's how you know it's good!

Combine all ingredients (starting with ½ avocado) in a food processor or blender and puree until smooth, stopping to scrape sides as necessary. Taste, adding more onion, garlic, Worcestershire sauce, hot sauce, lime, etc. to taste. For a richer, more guacamole-like flavor, puree in the remaining avocado.

PER SERVING
(1 TBSP, WITH ½ AVOCADO)

Calories	27
Fat	1.3g
Carbs	3.1g
Fiber	1.3g
Sugars	1.1g
Protein	0.9g
WW Points	1

MAKES 1 CUP

- ½ –1 avocado
- 1 c peas (thawed, if frozen)
- 1 tbsp onion flakes
- 1 tsp garlic powder
- 1 tsp Vegan Worcestershire Sauce (pg. 266)
- hot sauce
- juice of 1–2 lime slices
- cilantro (optional)
- sea salt
- ½ tsp ground cumin
- 1 tbsp nondairy milk

baked potato samosas

PER SAMOSA

Calories	90
Fat	0.6g
Carbs	18.9g
Fiber	3.2g
Sugars	2g
Protein	3.1g
WW Points	2

SERVES 4

2 potatoes

3–4 tbsp nondairy milk

¾ tsp yellow curry powder

½ tsp onion powder

½ tsp garlic powder

¼ – ¾ tsp garam masala

¼ tsp ground coriander

1 tsp prepared yellow mustard

cayenne (optional)

juice of 2 lemon wedges

½ c peas (thawed, if using frozen)

cilantro (garnish)

Chef's Note For some heat, you can add more cayenne to taste or 1–3 tbsp minced green chilies (canned).

When I was writing this cookbook, my Dad ("Papa Herbivore") e-mailed me, "I stopped @ an Indian booth and got a samosa. It was *so* good. Maybe you could make a recipe for your new cookbook." (My parents have turned into quite the foodies since going plant-based!) Knowing a samosa is usually fried, I thought about trying to bake them, but I'm pretty lazy with my cooking so even that seemed like too much work. That's when my Dad put the thought in my head to leave it all in the potato. Ah, yes—perfection!

Preheat oven to 400°F. Wrap potatoes in foil and bake for 1 hour. Let cool, then slice in half. Scoop out potato flesh, but leave some around the skin so it stays sturdy (don't scoop it clean). Transfer your scooped out potato flesh to a mixing bowl and mash with a potato masher or beaters, adding nondairy milk as necessary to get the right consistency. Add curry powder, onion powder, garlic powder, ¼ tsp garam masala, ground coriander, mustard, a light dash of cayenne, plus lemon juice, and stir or mix to combine. Taste, adding more garam masala, ground coriander, or curry powder to taste, ¼ tsp at a time (all blends are a little different in terms of potency). Add salt to taste. Stir in peas, then scoop mixture back into potato shells. Bake for another 5–10 minutes until just thoroughly warm. Garnish with cilantro before serving.

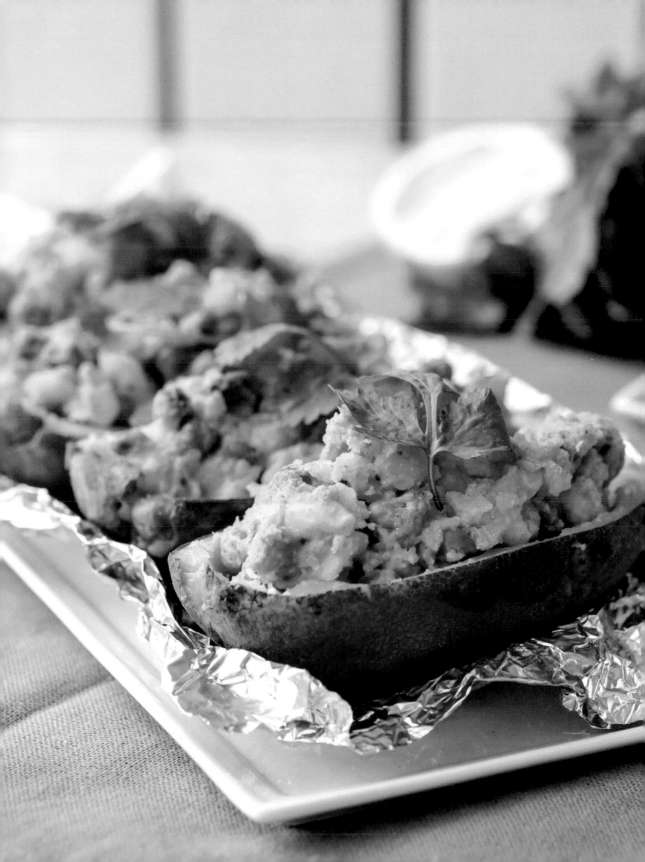

PER SERVING

CHICKPEA CHEESE SPREAD (1 TBSP) /
QUICK NACHO SAUCE (5 TBSP)

Calories 25/83
Fat. 0.3g/1.9g
Carbs 3.7g/11.7g
Fiber 1.1g/4.2g
Sugars. 0g/0.8g
Protein 1.8g/7.2g
WW Points 1/2

MAKES 1¼ CUPS

1 c cooked chickpeas
1–2 tbsp yellow miso
2 tbsp plus 1 tsp
 nutritional yeast
½ tsp onion powder
½ tsp garlic powder
3–4 tbsp vegetable broth
 juice of 1 lemon
 wedge

SERVES 4

1 c nondairy milk
⅓ c nutritional yeast
1½ tbsp cornstarch
1½ tbsp tomato paste
½ tsp onion powder
½ tsp garlic powder
½ tsp chili powder
½ tsp ground cumin
¼ tsp paprika or
 smoked paprika
1 tbsp yellow miso

chickpea "cheese" spread

This "cheese" spread is great on top of crackers or slipped into a sandwich. Since the base is chickpeas, it's a great low-fat and lower calorie alternative to nut-based vegan cheeses.

In a small food processor, combine all ingredients (starting with 1 tbsp miso) and whiz until smooth, adding broth as necessary to achieve the right consistency. Taste, adding more miso, nutritional yeast, or lemon to taste (all misos are a bit different in strength).

quick nacho sauce

I'm always tweaking my "cheese" sauce recipes and this is my favorite variation yet. It comes together about as fast as you can whisk and heat and it's a great way to jazz up a meal that needs a little something extra. You'll be pouring it on everything before you know it!

Whisk all ingredients except miso together in a saucepan and bring to a near-boil. Reduce heat to medium and allow sauce to thicken, stirring constantly. Add miso, stir again, and serve.

roasted chickpeas

If you love to snack on nuts, you'll love these crunchy chickpeas. They're a low-fat but still protein-packed alternative to nuts and they're crazy addictive! I tend to eat these chickpeas as a snack but they're great on salads, too!

Preheat oven to 400°F. Line a cookie sheet with parchment paper. Toss damp chickpeas with spices until well coated. Place on cookie sheet in a single layer and bake for 10 minutes. Give the tray a good shake so the chickpeas rotate and bake another 10 minutes. Bake another 5–10 minutes or until chickpeas are golden and crispy to your liking.

PER SERVING
(ABOUT ¼ CUP)

Calories 114
Fat. 0.8g
Carbs 18.4g
Fiber 4.4g
Sugars. 0g
Protein 6.2g
WW Points 2

SERVES 4

1 15-oz can chickpeas, drained and rinsed

spices (such as ground cumin, chili powder with a little cayenne, garlic salt, garam masala, a little chipotle, etc.)

tofu jerky

1 lb extra-firm tofu, pressed

MARINADE

¼ c low-sodium soy sauce or gluten-free tamari

¼ c vegetable broth

1 tbsp pure maple syrup

1–2 tsp liquid smoke

1 tsp onion powder

1 tsp garlic powder

¼ tsp smoked paprika

2–3 tbsp barbecue sauce

Chef's Note Disclaimer: Because not all of the marinade ingredients are absorbed by the tofu, it is hard to know the exact nutritional analysis of this recipe.

I'm slightly embarrassed to admit how much I liked jerky before I was plant-based. Let's just say one Christmas someone gave me a giant box of Slim Jims and it was my favorite gift. As you might imagine, I also love the commercial vegan versions of jerky, but I am sometimes put off by the ingredients list. This led me to wonder if I could make my own jerky from tofu. . . YES.

Press tofu for about 20 minutes, pat dry, cut into 12 strips (jerky size), and place in a Ziploc bag. Whisk marinade ingredients together and pour over tofu. Close bag and flip it over a few times so the marinade coats the tofu. Let marinate overnight, turning the bag over if you can (I turn mine over every time I go into the fridge). Preheat oven to 350°F. Line a cookie sheet with parchment paper. Place marinated tofu on prepared sheet (discard excess marinade) and bake 10 minutes. Flip over and bake 10 more minutes. Continue to cook until the tofu is dark brown and firm, but be careful not to burn. (I'm generally done after 35–40 minutes.)

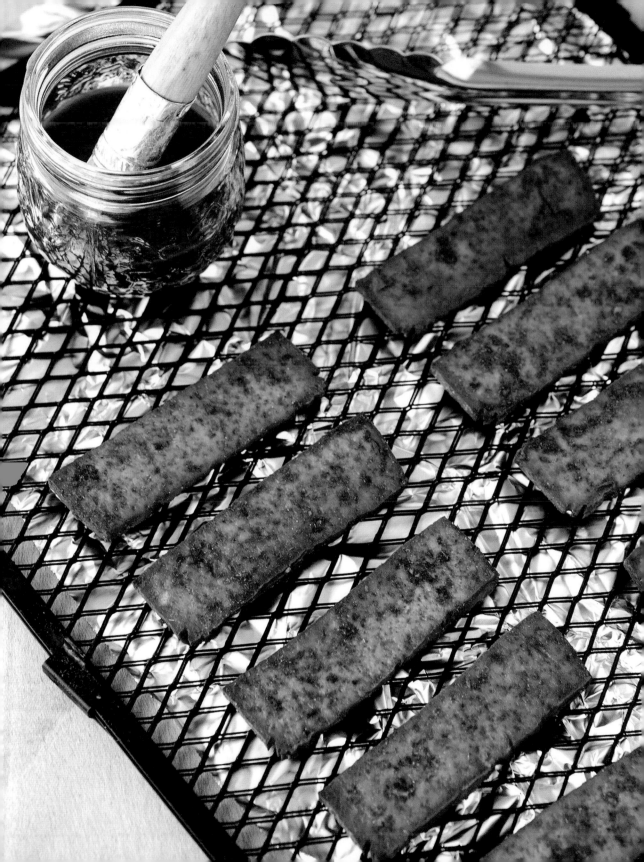

THE UTOPIA PARADOX

It would be ideal if we had a buffet of healthy, wholesome foods to choose from in every location and situation in life, but sometimes our only option is to select the best choice from what's in front of us. I call this the Utopia Paradox.

GOOD VS. BAD

So often, fans and 7-Day Meal Plan users ask me about "bad" foods. They'll say something like, "Is chocolate bad?" or "Is coffee bad?" or "How bad is sugar?"

I try not to associate "good" and "bad" with food choices or behaviors because I don't find that to be beneficial for me or my relationship with food, diet, life, etc. If I tell myself something is "bad" or eating it is "bad," I'll feel bad if I do eat it. I should be encouraging myself to make good choices, not berating myself when I slip up or make a less-than-perfect choice.

Of course, there are some clear villains—hydrogenated oils, high-fructose corn syrup, etc.—but generally speaking, I look at food on an overarching "healthy" scale and find that that allows me to make the best choices while also feeling good about them. For example, I don't consider white rice bad, but I recognize it's not as healthy as brown rice, which is "better." Similarly, I know white pasta is not as healthy as whole-wheat or brown rice pasta, and that brown rice pasta is not as healthy as a whole grain (like brown rice itself). See the difference?

If I'm at a restaurant and the only choice is white rice, I'm not going to tell myself it's bad or that I'm bad if I eat it. If there's brown rice, I'll get

> I should be encouraging myself to make good choices, not berating myself when I slip up or make a less-than-perfect choice.

brown rice, but sometimes I just have to do the best that I can. After all, white rice with steamed vegetables is still a whole lot better than deep-fried spring rolls!

This system allows you to account for the situation you're in. A few days ago I was in an airport and while I'd have loved to have found a whole-wheat bagel, the options were white bagels, cheese-covered bagels, or multigrain bagels (basically white bread with a tan). Still, a multigrain bagel is a far better choice than the others, and so I loaded it up with mustard and vegetables to make a sandwich that was light years healthier than the Big Mac sold across the terminal. I'm not "bad" because I ate white bread. My sandwich wasn't "bad" either; it just wasn't *ideal*—that is, the best possible choice if you had access to all of food utopia.

ORGANIC VS. NOT ORGANIC

Identifying the best choice is also how I deal with organic versus not organic. I can't always find an organic option and sometimes the organic option is too far out of my price range or it's flown in from somewhere so far away that I can't justify it over the more conventional local item. I don't look at the conventional apple and tell myself it's bad for me. I recognize that it's not ideal, but like I said, I have to do the best I can, and a conventional apple is still way better than organic potato chips.

So when looking at your food choices, ask yourself what's the better choice from the options in front of you, not from utopia.

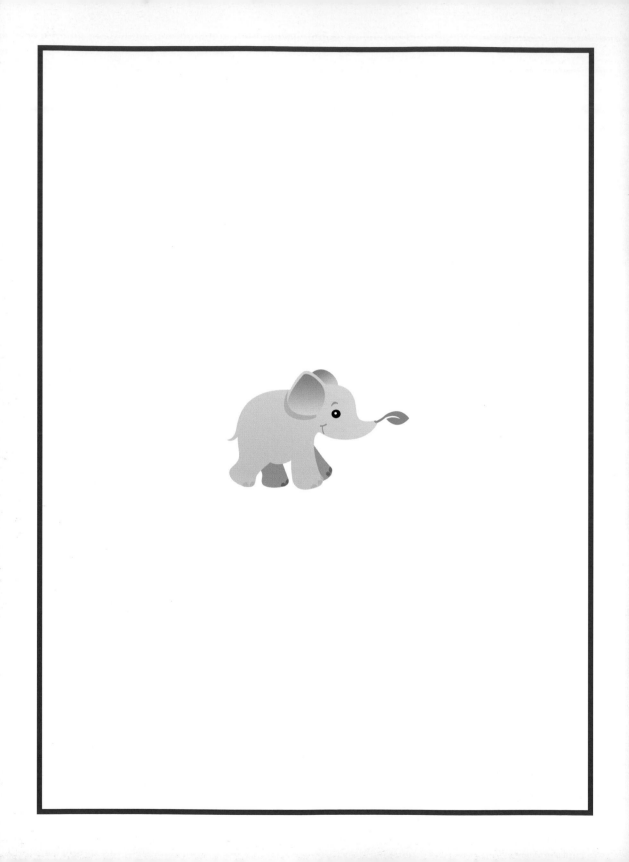

desserts

chocolate chip cookies

PER COOKIE

Calories 61
Fat 0.7g
Carbs 12.5g
Fiber 1.0g
Sugars 6.2g
Protein 1.0g
WW Points 2

MAKES 16

- ⅓ c unsweetened applesauce
- ½ c light brown sugar
- 1 tsp vanilla extract
- ¼ c nondairy milk
- 1 c whole-wheat pastry flour
- 1 tsp baking powder
- ¼ tsp fine salt
- 1 tbsp cornstarch
- few dashes of ground cinnamon
- ½ c vegan chocolate chips

Chef's Note For a firmer cookie, work a fresh banana into the flour (crumble it in until you have clumps). If your banana is ripe, reduce sugar.

These are the best low-fat chocolate chip cookies you'll ever eat! They're ridiculously addictive fresh out of the oven. You've been warned.

Preheat oven to 350°F. Grease cookie sheet or line with parchment paper. In a large bowl, combine applesauce, sugar, vanilla extract, and nondairy milk. In a small bowl, whisk flour, baking powder, salt, cornstarch, and ground cinnamon together. Transfer the dry mixture into the wet mixture in three batches. Stir until almost combined. Fold in chips. Drop spoonfuls on cookie sheet and bake for 7–10 minutes for a soft and light cookie or a few minutes more for a firmer cookie, being careful not to burn.

VARIATION

Double Chocolate Chip Cookies: Replace 2 tbsp of flour with 2 tbsp of unsweetened cocoa.

molasses cake

If you loved the Tortuga Rum Cake in *Everyday Happy Herbivore*, you'll love this old-fashioned virgin cousin. It's a rich, moist cake with a just a hint of spice and sweetness.

Preheat oven to 350°F. Set aside a square 8-inch non-stick cake pan or round springform pan. In a mixing bowl, whisk flours, baking powder, baking soda, salt (if using), allspice (reduce to ¾ tsp if your allspice is very strong), and brown sugar until well combined. Add remaining ingredients through nondairy milk and stir until just combined (it'll be pretty wet). Pour batter into cake pan and bake 35–40 minutes. Dust with powdered sugar if desired before serving.

PER PIECE

Calories	167
Fat	1.2g
Carbs	36.3g
Fiber	1.6g
Sugars	16.3g
Protein	2.9g
WW Points	4

SERVES 9

- 1 c oat flour (see Chef's Note)
- 1 c white whole-wheat flour
- 1 tsp baking powder
- ½ tsp baking soda
- pinch of salt (optional)
- 1 tsp allspice
- ⅔ c brown sugar
- ¼ c molasses (see chef's note)
- ¼ c applesauce
- 1 tsp vanilla extract
- 1 c nondairy milk
- powdered sugar (garnish)

Chef's Notes

» To make oat flour, pulverize oats in a blender.

» Do not use blackstrap molasses in this recipe.

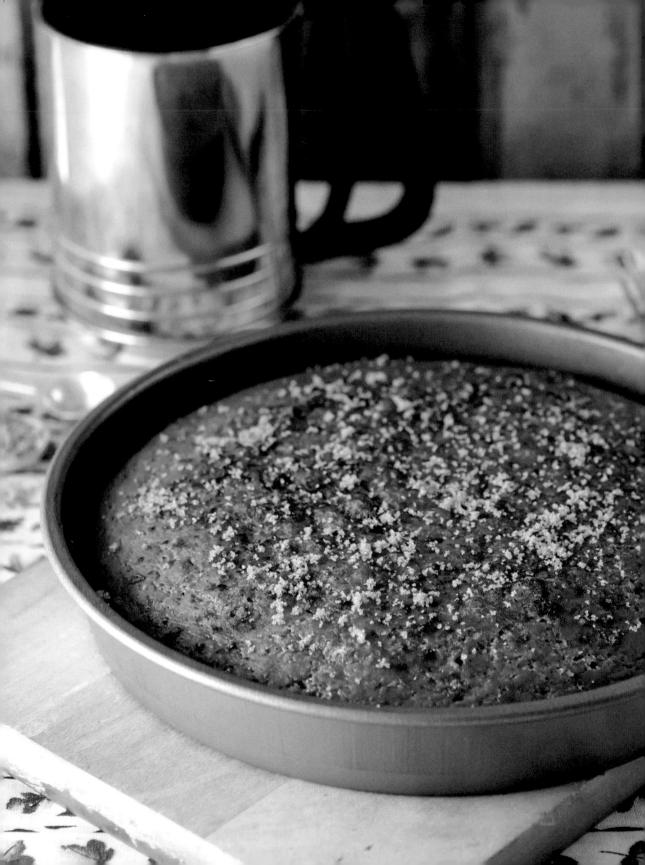

spice cake surprise

When I started writing this cookbook, my dad pulled out an old church collaborative cookbook from the 1990s and sent me a few ideas—old recipes I could make over, he said. The one that stuck out the most was Tomato Soup Cake. I just couldn't wrap my head around the idea of dumping a can of soup into a box cake mix but eventually curiosity got the best of me and I developed this recipe. I'm slightly ashamed to say it's one of my absolute favorite cakes now. Who knew tomato sauce rocked a cake? Surprise!

Preheat oven to 350°F. Grease a cake pan or line with parchment paper or use nonstick bakeware. In a mixing bowl, whisk flour, baking soda, baking powder, sugar, and pumpkin pie spice together (for a very spiced cake, you can add more pumpkin pie spice). Stir in tomato sauce, applesauce, and water, adding an extra splash of water if necessary. Pour into prepared pan and sprinkle generously with brown sugar and pumpkin pie spice. Bake 20–30 minutes, or until it springs back to the touch and a toothpick inserted in the center comes out clean.

PER SLICE

Calories 114
Fat 0.4g
Carbs 25.9g
Fiber 2.5g
Sugars 11.9g
Protein 3g
WW Points 3

SERVES 9

- 1½ c white whole-wheat flour
- 1 tsp baking soda
- ½ tsp baking powder
- ⅓ –½ c raw sugar
- 1 tsp pumpkin pie spice
- 1 8-oz can tomato sauce
- 5 tbsp unsweetened applesauce
- ¼ c water
- brown sugar

Chef's Note I use no-salt-added tomato sauce, but regular tomato sauce should work fine.

chocolate cake

PER SERVING

Calories	128
Fat	2.3g
Carbs	25.2g
Fiber	2.9g
Sugars	11.9g
Protein	3.2g
WW Points	3

SERVES 9

1¼ c white whole-wheat flour

¼ c unsweetened cocoa

1 tsp baking soda

½ tsp baking powder

pinch salt (optional)

½ c brown sugar

1 c nondairy milk (plain or chocolate)

6 tbsp unsweetened applesauce

2 tbsp balsamic vinegar

1 tsp chocolate or vanilla extract

¼ c vegan chocolate chips

Balsamic vinegar is the secret to chocolate cake. (You'll see!) This cake is cheap, quick, and sure to please. I also like to omit the chips and spread a thick layer of Chocolate Surprise Frosting on top.

Preheat oven to 375°F. Set aside an 8-inch square nonstick cake pan or round springform pan. In a mixing bowl, whisk flour, cocoa, baking soda, baking powder, and salt (if using) together. Add sugar, nondairy milk, applesauce, balsamic vinegar, and extract, stirring until just combined. Transfer batter to your pan and sprinkle with chocolate chips. Bake 20–30 minutes, until it springs back to the touch and a toothpick inserted in the center comes out clean.

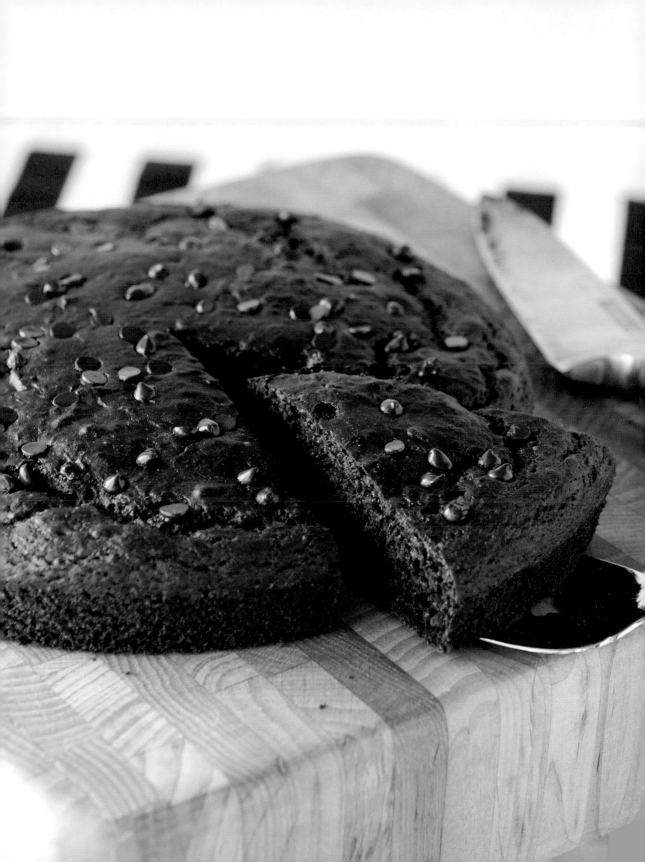

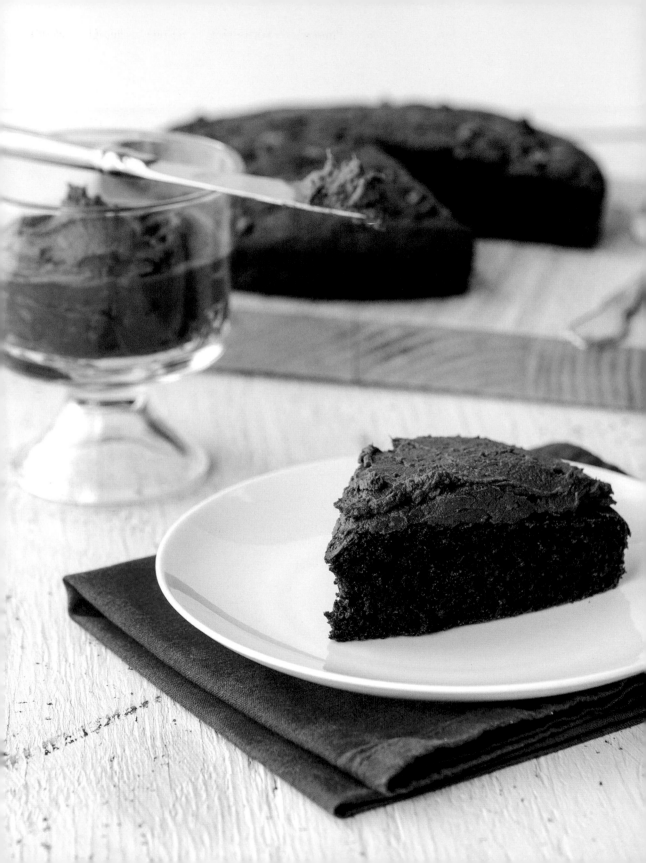

✓ SOY-FREE ✓ GLUTEN-FREE ✓ FAT-FREE ✓ BUDGET ✓ PANTRY

chocolate surprise frosting

This frosting is made from a sweet potato—surprise! I originally developed this recipe to replace traditional chocolate frosting for cakes and cupcakes, but my testers started using it as a chocolate hazelnut spread replacement on their toast, bagels, you name it, too! Frost away my friends, frost away! (P. S. This frosting has no added sugar or fat, so it's totally okay to go at it with a spoon!)

Combine sweet potato with 2 dates and 1 tbsp cocoa in a mini food processor and whiz until combined and smooth and shiny in appearance. Taste, adding more dates or cocoa as desired. (I start with 2 dates and 1 tbsp cocoa, then typically increase to 3 dates and 2 tbsp cocoa—but for a rich, deep dark chocolate taste, you'll probably want to go up to 3 tbsp cocoa.)

PER 1 TBSP
(3 DATES, 2 TBSP COCOA)

Calories	12
Fat	0.1g
Carbs	3g
Fiber	0.6g
Sugars	1.5g
Protein	0.3g
WW Points	0

MAKES 1 CUP

1 c mashed sweet potato (no skin)

2–3 soaked dates

1–3 tbsp unsweetened cocoa

Chef's Notes

» I typically steam my sweet potatoes for quickness, but roasting the potato in the oven would make it much sweeter.

» Soak dates overnight or in *hot* water for 10 minutes.

PER SERVING
(WITH BLUEBERRIES)

Calories 97
Fat. 0.8g
Carbs 22.1g
Fiber 1.8g
Sugars. 11.6g
Protein 1.5g
WW Points 3

SERVES 6

⅓ c white whole-wheat
   flour

⅓ c instant oats

1 tsp baking powder

½ tsp baking soda
   ground cinnamon

3 tbsp pure maple
   syrup or agave nectar

3 tbsp unsweetened
   applesauce

⅔ c nondairy milk

2 c blueberries, or
   other berries, divided

cobbler

My husband is Southern and grew up eating all kinds of cobblers—blackberry cobbler, peach cobbler, blueberry cobbler. Cobbler wasn't something I grew up with, but I certainly helped myself to many servings of cobblers when I lived in Charleston, South Carolina, and can thus appreciate why my husband is always longing for them. I've been tinkering with my mother-in-law's cobbler recipe for a while now, trying to catch the same texture and consistency, but without the butter and white flour. I find oats help give this cobbler a sturdy structure while also making it more filling.

Preheat oven to 350°F and set aside glass pie dish. In a bowl, whisk flour, oats, baking powder, baking soda, and a few dashes of ground cinnamon together until combined. Add maple syrup, applesauce, and nondairy milk, and stir again. Fold half the berries into the batter then pour batter into the pie dish. Add remaining berries on top. Let cobbler rest for a few minutes if you can, then bake 30–40 minutes, until firm to the touch, lightly brown in color, and cooked through.

VARIATION

Use lemon zest instead of ground cinnamon.

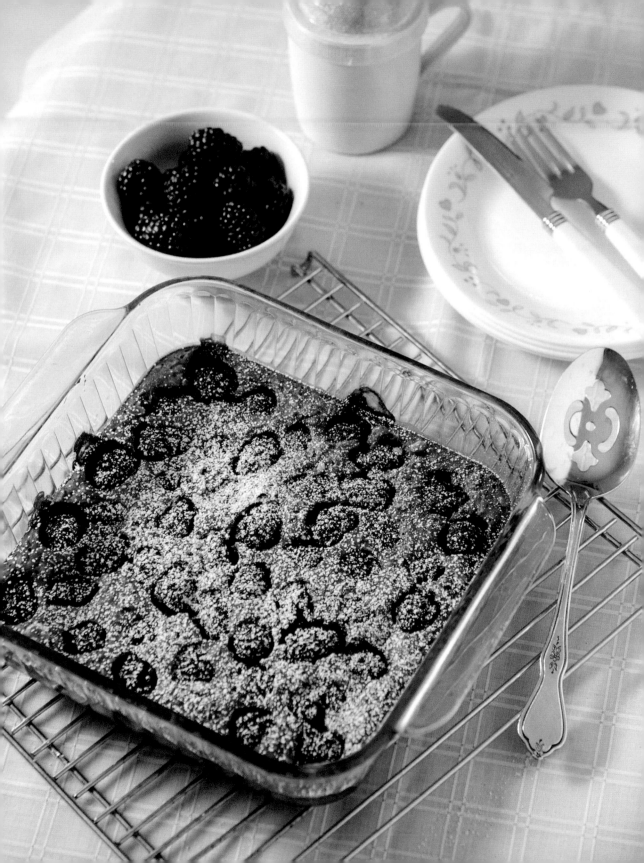

PER BALL

Calories	39
Fat	1g
Carbs	6.2g
Fiber	1.8g
Sugars	1.4g
Protein	2g
WW Points	1

MAKES 10

- 1 c cooked white beans
- 1 tbsp smooth peanut butter
- 1 tbsp pure maple syrup
- 2 tbsp unsweetened cocoa

Chef's Notes

» Any white beans, such as navy, cannellini, or butter bean, will work in this recipe.

» If you want to get all fancy pants, roll crushed vegan chocolate chips or nut pieces into the balls.

dark chocolate truffles

Only 39 calories a pop.

Combine all ingredients in food processor and allow motor to run. Stop to scrape the sides as necessary, until you have a smooth and homogenous mixture. Taste, adding another 1 tbsp maple syrup for a sweeter chocolate (you don't want it to get too wet though). The "batter" should be thick and pliable. Pick off 10 pieces and roll into bouncy bite–size balls.

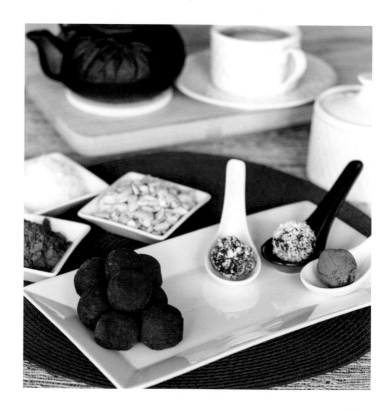

brownies

Don't get me wrong, I love my Internet-famous Black Bean Brownies, but I wanted to create a brownie recipe that was a little more like a traditional brownie. Mmm, yes! More chocolate, please!

Preheat oven to 350°F. Set aside an 8-inch square nonstick pan. In a food processor or blender, combine tofu with 1 tbsp nondairy milk, extract, vinegar, and agave nectar, whizzing until smooth (adding another 1 tbsp nondairy milk if necessary to get it to combine), and set aside. In a mixing bowl, whisk flour, baking soda, cocoa, and sugar together. Add tofu mixture in and stir to combine, adding another 1–2 tbsp nondairy milk (the batter should be thick and glossy, but no flour dusting). Stir in chocolate chips. Transfer batter to your pan and bake 15–20 minutes, until firm to the touch and starting to crack slightly.

PER SERVING

Calories	128
Fat	2.3g
Carbs	25.2g
Fiber	2.9g
Sugars	11.9g
Protein	3.2g
WW Points	3

SERVES 9

- 1 pkg Mori-Nu tofu (firm or extra-firm)
- 2–3 tbsp nondairy milk (plain, chocolate, or vanilla), divided
- ½ tsp vanilla or chocolate extract
- 1 tbsp balsamic vinegar
- ¼ c agave nectar
- ¾ c white whole-wheat flour
- 1 tsp baking soda
- 6 tbsp unsweetened cocoa
- 2 tbsp brown sugar
- ½ –1 c vegan chocolate chips

Chef's Note Mori-Nu is a shelf-stable tofu. While other brands exist, Mori-Nu is the most common and available at most supermarkets, usually in the Asian section. You can also substitute 12.3 oz silken tofu (note silken is usually sold in 12–16-oz packages, so you will need to adjust).

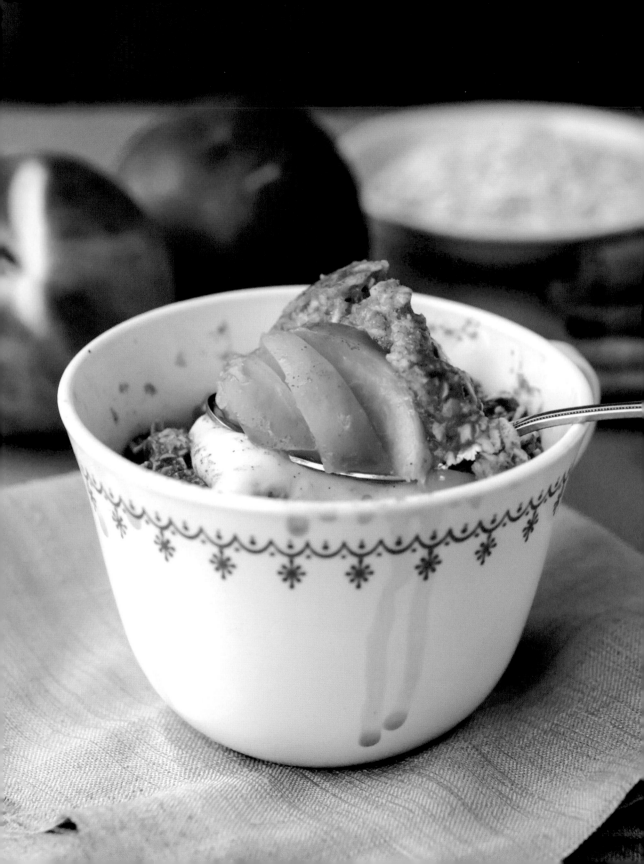

microwave peach cobbler

After the success of the Mug Cake in *Everyday Happy Herbivore* I wondered if I could make a pie or cobbler in a mug in my microwave. Still working on the pie, but this cobbler rocks!

Place peaches in your mug and set aside for a few seconds to thaw peaches if they're frozen. In a small bowl, whisk flour, instant oats, rolled oats (if you want a slightly oat-y cobbler), brown sugar, and a few dashes of ground cinnamon (about ⅛ tsp), and a light dash or two ground nutmeg, until combined. Then stir in nondairy milk. Place the oat mixture on top of the peaches and microwave 1–2 minutes, until the oat topping has cooked and looks a little like oatmeal. Top with yogurt and serve.

PER COBBLER

Calories	137
Fat	1.2g
Carbs	29.2g
Fiber	2.4g
Sugars	18.2g
Protein	3.4g
WW Points	4

SINGLE SERVING

- 1 peach, sliced (about 1½ cups)
- 1 tbsp white whole-wheat flour
- 2 tbsp instant oats
- 1 tbsp rolled oats (optional)
- 1–2 tbsp brown sugar
    ground cinnamon
    ground nutmeg
- 1–2 tbsp nondairy milk (more with fresh peaches; frozen peaches are juicier)
- 1–2 tbsp vanilla vegan yogurt

PER SERVING
WITHOUT COCOA/WITH COCOA (1 TSP)

Calories 112/118
Fat. 0.8g/1.1g
Carbs 27.5g/29g
Fiber 3.3g/4.1g
Sugars. 14.5g/14.6g
Protein 1.4g/1.9g
WW Points 3

SERVES 2

2 frozen bananas
¼ c nondairy milk
¼ tsp vanilla extract
¼ tsp ground cinnamon

banana ice cream

This banana-based ice cream made its debut in my second cookbook, *Everyday Happy Herbivore*, but it deserves a spot in this book, too! It's so easy to make and the number-one reason why I always have frozen bananas in my freezer. Anytime the craving for rich and creamy ice cream hits, make this instead! P.S. I love (love!) topping this ice cream off with chocolate balsamic vinegar. (I'm not crazy, I swear!)

Place all ingredients together in a food processor and allow the motor to run until the mixture is smooth and creamy. Stop and break up large clumps with a spatula as needed.

VARIATION

I like to add 1–2 tbsp unsweetened cocoa for a chocolate version.

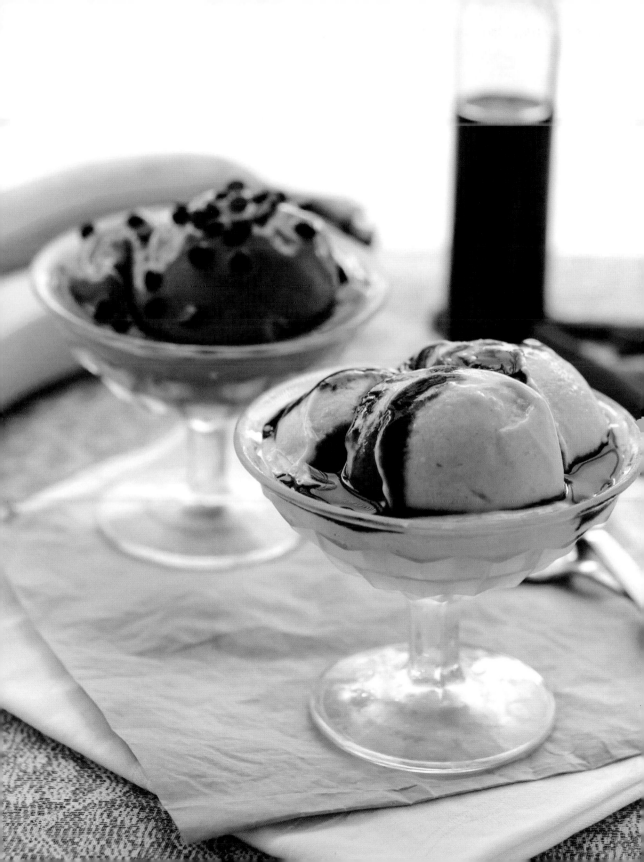

sweet potato ice cream

My friend Natala turned me on to making "ice cream" from sweet potatoes. It's not the most conventional ice cream around, but it's healthy and a great way to use up leftover sweet potatoes.

PER SERVING

Calories	103
Fat	0.2g
Carbs	23.6g
Fiber	3.8g
Sugars	7.4g
Protein	2.3g
WW Points	3

SERVES 2

2 sweet potatoes

nondairy milk

spices (e.g., ground cinnamon or pumpkin pie spice; optional)

sweetener (e.g., pure maple syrup; optional)

Chef's Notes

» While you can boil, steam, or microwave your potatoes, I find baking them makes them sweeter so no additional sweetener is required.

» My friend Chrysanthe stops midway in the process when the sweet potatoes are ground up into little frozen balls in the blender— it's her healthy substitute for Dippin' Dots.

Preheat oven to 350°F. Stab potatoes with a fork, wrap in foil, and roast in the oven for about 45 minutes or until fork-tender and soft. Once soft, peel away skin (if desired) and cube. Place cubes in ice cube tray slots or on a cookie sheet lined with parchment paper and freeze. Once frozen, you can put all the pieces in a plastic bag or airtight container. (If you do not freeze the pieces individually, they will freeze into a big blob.)

Place frozen sweet potatoes in a food processor (or a strong blender) and cream into an ice cream, adding nondairy milk as required to get the right consistency. You can also add spices or sweetener to taste and mix again. Serve immediately.

tofu ice cream

This basic recipe was developed by the chefs at Goodbaker Gourmet, a vegan baking mix company that sadly was closed by the owner. I found their tofu ice cream recipe online several years ago and have been playing with it ever since to create all sorts of ice cream flavors like vanilla, chocolate, banana, cinnamon, strawberry, and blueberry!

Combine all ingredients in a blender and whiz until smooth. Transfer mixture to an ice cream machine and allow the machine to run until ice cream has formed, about 30 minutes. Serve immediately.

PER SERVING

Calories	103
Fat	3.1g
Carbs	12.7g
Sugars	10g
Fiber	0g
Protein	6.3g
WW Points	3

SERVES 4

- 12 oz soft or silken tofu (such as Mori-Nu)
- 1 c nondairy milk
- 3 tbsp pure maple syrup
- flavorings (optional) (see Chef's Note)

Chef's Note For flavors, add in an extract, such as vanilla (1½–2 tsp; adds 6 calories), or frozen fruit, such as 2 ripe bananas (adds 53 calories) or 18 strawberries (adds 17 calories). The possibilities are endless!

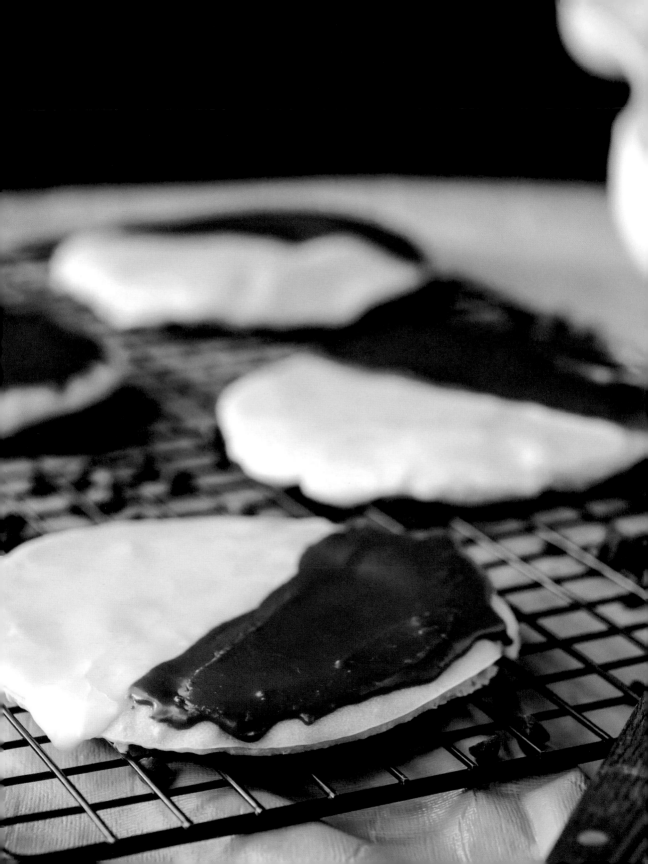

black & white cookies

For years I've wanted to develop a recipe for this New York City staple but the pressure to re-create my all-time favorite cookie was intense! I decided to tackle it with this cookbook and. . . yes—1,000 times, yes. By the way, while most people say these deli cookies are best eaten day-of and fresh, I like them a day old!

Preheat oven to 350°F. Line a cookie sheet with parchment paper and set aside. In a mixing bowl, whisk flour, cornstarch, baking powder, and salt together. Add extract, zest, ½ cup nondairy milk, and vegan yogurt, and stir to combine. Add another 1–2 tbsp nondairy milk. (It should resemble pancake batter.)

Scoop up ¼-cup batter and pour it onto the sheet, leaving room for it to spread. Repeat for 6 total cookies. Bake 10–15 minutes, until the cookies are golden and spring back to the touch. Allow to cool completely.

Meanwhile, combine confectioner's sugar with *hot* water and almond extract, whisking vigorously. Whisk in 1 tsp more water if necessary. You don't want it too runny; it should be shiny and white. Flip cookies over and paint half of each cookie white with a spatula. Heat 1–2 tbsp chocolate chips in a microwave for a few seconds, until melted—careful not to burn. Whisk into leftover icing. It'll be a nice coffee-with-cream color. Use spatula to paint the other side of the cookies "black." Allow to cool completely.

PER COOKIE
(LARGE)

Calories 184
Fat. 1.1g
Carbs 39.6g
Fiber 0.8g
Sugars. 21.5g
Protein 2.9g
WW Points 5

MAKES 6

1 c white whole-wheat flour
1 tbsp cornstarch
1 tsp baking powder
    pinch salt
1 tsp vanilla extract
1½ tsp lemon zest
½ c plus 1–2 tbsp nondairy milk
¼ c vegan yogurt (plain or vanilla)

ICING

1 c confectioner's sugar
1 tbsp boiling hot water
1 tsp almond extract
1–2 tbsp vegan chocolate chips

Chef's Note For smaller cookies, use a 2-tbsp measuring spoon to scoop the batter and bake a few minutes less. Bonus: The mini size is only 93 calories *with* frosting!

PER CUPCAKE
(WITH JAM TOPPING)

Calories 140
Fat 0.6g
Carbs 34.2g
Fiber 2.3g
Sugars 13.5g
Protein 3.1g
WW Points 4

SINGLE SERVING

- 3 tbsp white whole-wheat flour
- 1 tbsp raw sugar
- ¼ tsp baking powder
- ¼ tsp vanilla extract
- 1 tbsp nondairy milk
- 1 tbsp jam (e.g., strawberry)
- whole fresh berries or strawberry slices (garnish)

skinny cupcake

A cupcake for one! I top this cupcake with jam and fresh fruit (fresh raspberries or strawberry slices) but it's also delish with the Chocolate Surprise Frosting (pg. 227) and sprinkles!

Preheat oven or toaster oven to 350°F. Line a single muffin cup or a metal 1-cup measuring cup with a liner, or use a foil baking cup (e.g., Reynolds) that will stand on its own, or silicone cup, and set aside. In a small bowl, whisk flour, sugar, and baking powder together. Then stir in vanilla extract and non-dairy milk. Transfer batter to your muffin cup and bake 15–20 minutes, or until a toothpick inserted in the center comes out clean. Top with jam (that's your "icing") and fresh berries, if desired.

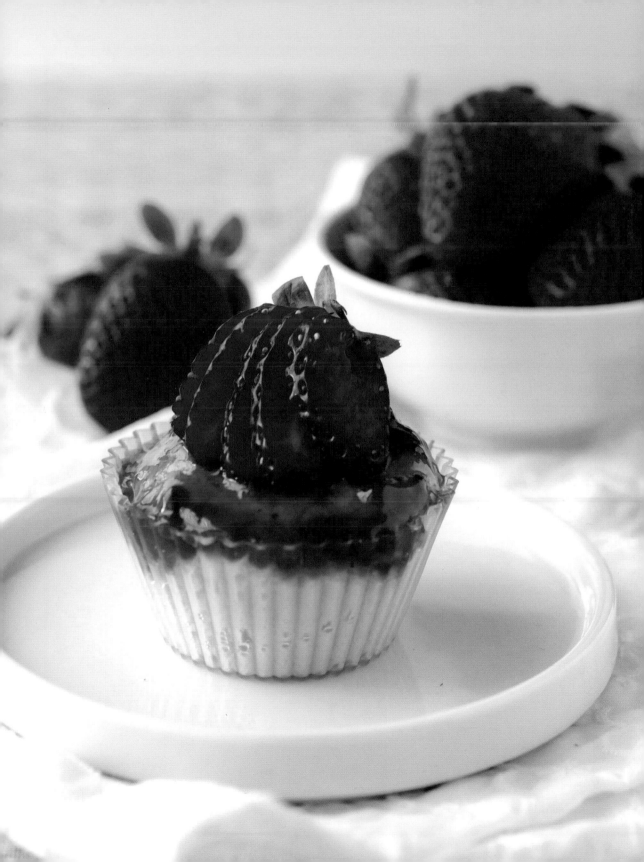

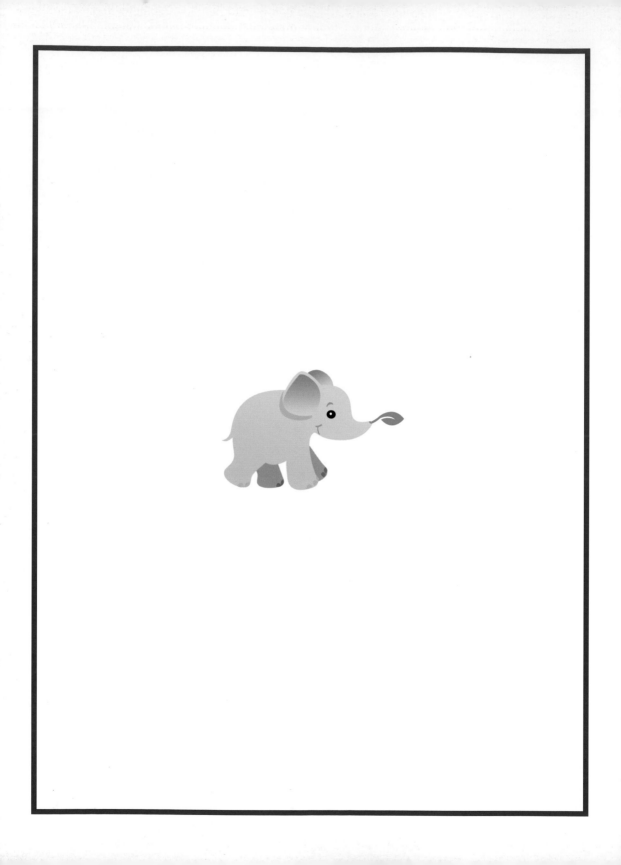

drinks

PER SERVING
(WITHOUT FRUIT SLICES)

Calories 70
Fat. 0.1g
Carbs 6.4g
Fiber 0g
Sugars. 4.4g
Protein 0.4g
WW Points 1

SINGLE SERVING

1 small orange

¼ c red wine (preferably chilled)

¼ c mixed-berry-flavored sparkling water

apple slice (optional)

orange slice (optional)

sangria spritzer

This is a lightened-up take on sangria. It's refreshing and has barely any alcohol at all—making it great for the punch bowl at parties. If you're looking for a more traditional sangria, check out my recipe in *Happy Herbivore Abroad* (I brought it back from Spain!).

Fill a highball glass (or just a tall, narrow drinking glass) with large ice cubes and a slice of orange and apple if using. Squeeze juice from the orange into the glass. Add wine, then sparking water. Stir, adding more water (or wine) as desired.

Chef's Note If you make a big pitcher of this, add a whole sliced apple, whole sliced orange, and a cinnamon stick or two.

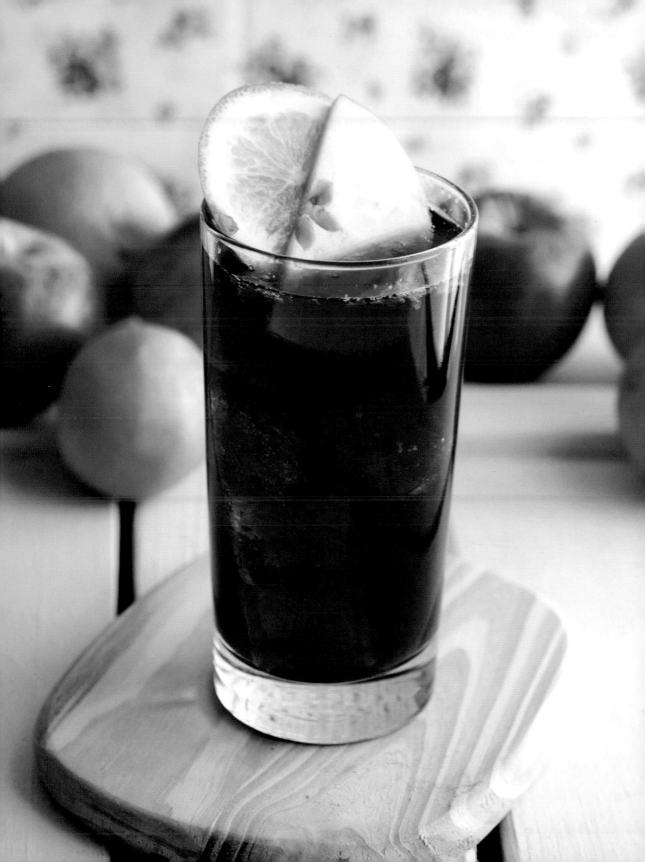

PER SERVING

Calories 107
Fat 2g
Carbs 22.9g
Fiber 2.8g
Sugars 15.1g
Protein 1.3g
WW Points 3

SINGLE SERVING

¾ c vanilla nondairy
   milk
1 frozen banana
   dash ground nutmeg
   dash cloves
¼ tsp ground cinnamon
   (garnish)

"eggnog"

A healthy version of the quintessential holiday drink!
Now you can really be merry!

Combine all ingredients in a blender and blend until
smooth. Garnish with ground cinnamon and serve.

overnight iced coffee

DIY iced coffee has become all the rage online—bloggers everywhere are making their own iced coffee to skip out on the coffee shop price tag and control the added milk and sugar. There seem to be two common methods: The first is brewing coffee, then just chilling it, but I find that makes for a too strong iced coffee with a slightly stale taste. This recipe is the second method. It's a touch more work, but tastes so much better. Plus you get about 5 cups, enough to power you through a couple of days or to invite some friends over for a cup o' joe.

In a pitcher or large container, combine water, ground coffee, and spices if you'd like an added flavor (careful not to exceed 2–3 tsp, depending on potency of your spices). Place a lid on your container to prevent odors from the fridge attaching to the coffee. Let set overnight in the fridge, giving it a good stir before bed.

   In the morning, strain through cheesecloth into another pitcher—this is your brew. Fill a mason jar (or glass) with ice and pour black coffee over the ice, leaving room for nondairy milk and sweetener (add to taste). The brew will last a few days in your fridge in an airtight container.

PER SERVING
(1 CUP)

Calories	2
Fat	0.1g
Carbs	0g
Fiber	0g
Sugars	0g
Protein	0.3g
WW Points	0

MAKES 5 CUPS

- **5 c water**
- **2.5 oz individual ground coffee packet**
- **spices (e.g., cinnamon stalk, ground cinnamon, ground ginger, vanilla bean, etc.; optional)**
- **ice**
- **nondairy milk (optional)**
- **sweetener (optional)**

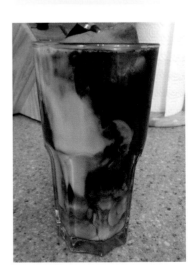

PER SERVING
WITH CALORIE-FREE COLA/
WITH REGULAR COLA

Calories	128/138
Fat	0g/0g
Carbs	12.1g/14.7g
Fiber	0g/0g
Sugars	11.1g/13.6g
Protein	0g/0g
WW Points	1

SINGLE SERVING

ice
1 oz vodka
1 oz Kahlúa
1 oz cola
1 oz Guinness

dublin

When I was in Ireland, I saw a drink on the menu called a "Black Russian from Dublin," which was described as a combination of vodka, Kahlúa, cola, and Guinness. It sounded, well, gross, and yet curiosity was killing me so I ordered one. Perhaps one of the best drinks I've ever had! I've since taken to calling it a "Dublin" and have all my friends hooked. Whenever I visit a bar that has Guinness on tap, I also teach the bartender how to make this drink. I'm that committed!

Fill a rocks/whisky glass with large ice cubes. Add the rest of the ingredients in order. Stir, if desired, and serve.

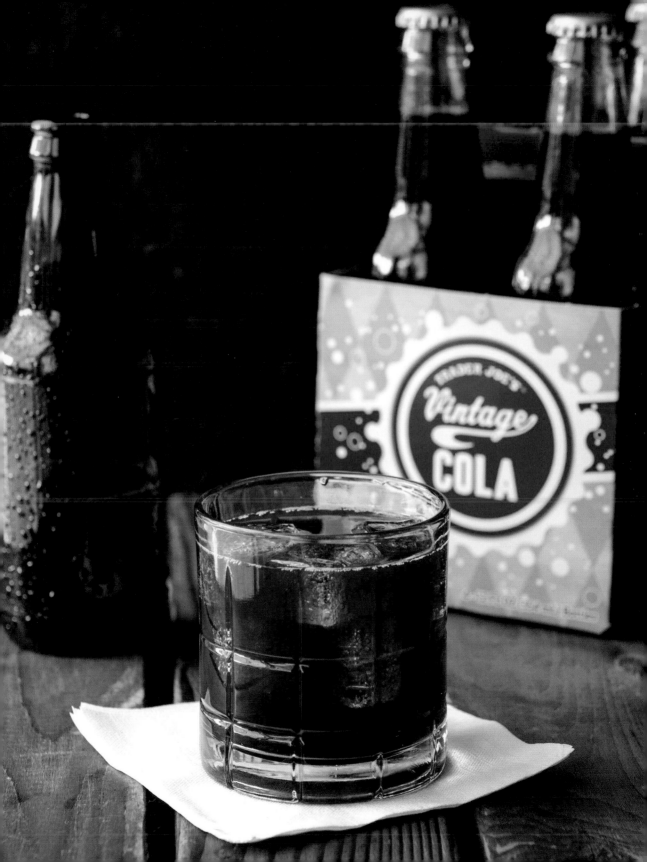

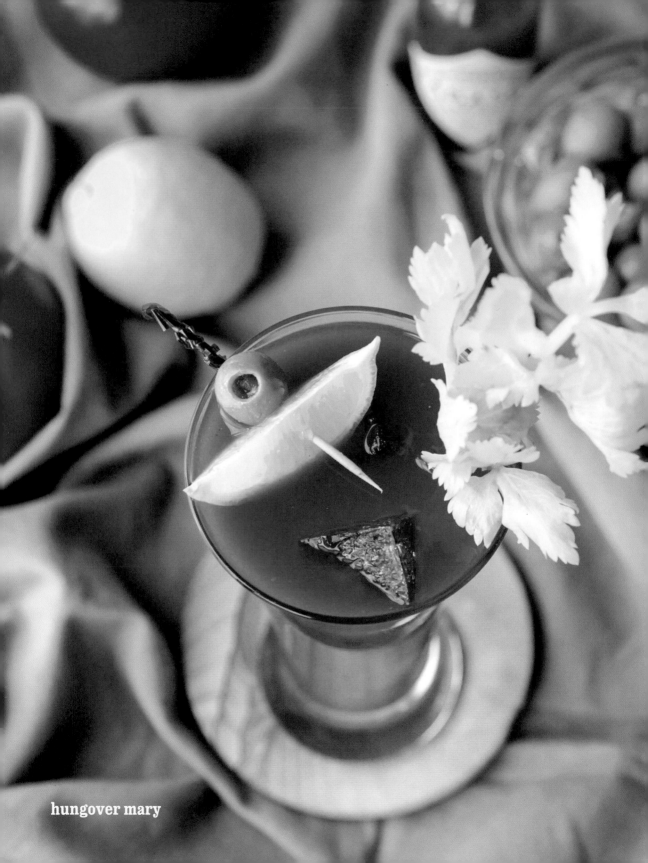

hungover mary

bloody mary mix

I love a good Bloody Mary and here's my DIY version. Most of the commercial Bloody Mary mixes are filled with scary ingredients, so I set out to create my own version using tomato sauce. It's so easy to make!

Whisk all ingredients together with 8 oz water (I fill the tomato sauce can with water). Taste, adding more hot sauce, Dijon, or spices as desired. (I like mine with a kick, so I tend to add another ½ tsp Dijon and black pepper.)

hungover mary

Fill a highball glass or tall, narrow drink glass with ice. Pour in vodka and Bloody Mary Mix, plus lime, lemon, green olives (if using), a splash of brine (if using), and then stir with the celery stalk.

Chef's Note I've also been served a pickle instead of celery and a green bean instead of celery (in British Columbia, Canada). Another option is to add in some brine from green olives.

PER SERVING
BLOODY MARY MIX / HUNGOVER MARY (WITHOUT GREEN OLIVES)

Calories	33/169
Fat	0.4g/0.8g
Carbs	6.9g/15.2g
Fiber	1.9g/4.1g
Sugars	5.1g/10.8g
Protein	1.8g/3.7g
WW Points	1/2

SERVES 2

- 8 oz tomato sauce
- 1 tbsp hot sauce
- 1½ tsp Dijon mustard
- 1½ tsp Vegan Worcestershire Sauce (pg. 266)
- ¼ tsp onion powder
- ¼ tsp garlic powder
- ¼ tsp black pepper
- salt (optional)
- celery seed (optional)

SERVES 2

- 1.5 oz vodka
- 1 serving Bloody Mary Mix
- 1 lime wedge
- 1 lemon wedge
- green olives (optional)
- celery stalk
- celery salt/black salt for the rim (optional)

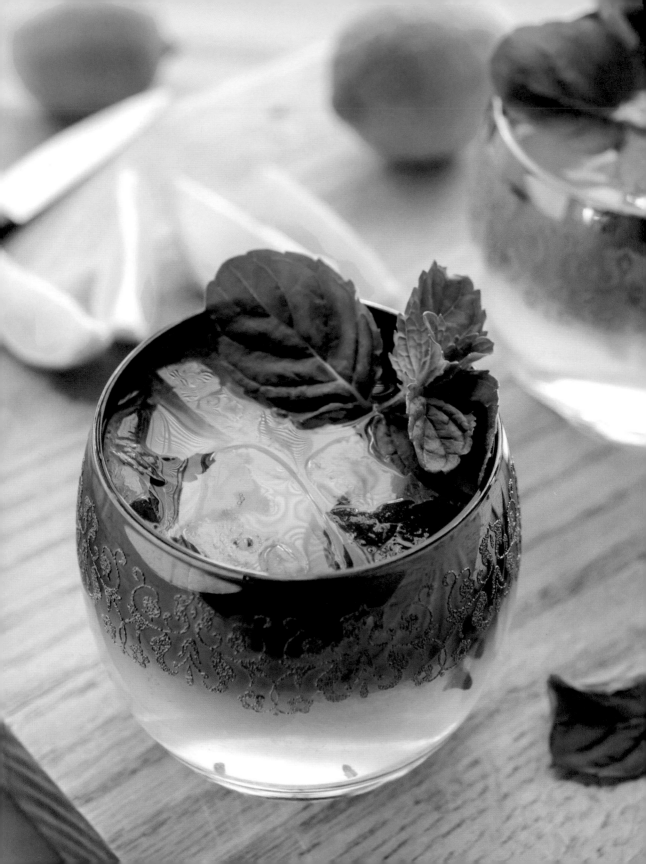

mojito

To cut calories in a mojito at the bar, ask for it unsweetened—no sugar or syrup. At home, you can add just a touch to your taste. The flavored water in this recipe also helps trick your tongue into thinking it's sweetened while adding a fun fizz.

Fill a rocks/whisky glass with 2–3 large ice cubes. Add rum (I like dark, but clear also works) and sparkling water. Squeeze lime juice into glass, then add lime wedges. Tear a handful of fresh mint and add to drink, plus a few drops of agave nectar or a pinch of brown sugar. Then pour into a beverage shaker and shake away. Taste, adding more lime, mint, sparkling water, or sweetener to taste. Garnish with a mint leaf or two and serve.

PER SERVING

Calories	112
Fat	0.1g
Carbs	3.3g
Fiber	1.2g
Sugars	0.8g
Protein	0.6g
WW Points	0

SINGLE SERVING

ice
1.5 oz rum
½ c lime-flavored sparking water
2 lime wedges
fresh mint (lots!)
agave nectar or brown sugar

PER SERVING
MINT MOCHA / HOT CHOCOLATE

Calories 167/135
Fat. 9.6g/4.8g
Carbs 17.5g/24.3g
Fiber 1.3g/3g
Sugars. 14.6g/19.1g
Protein 2.6g/2.4g
WW Points 4/4

SINGLE SERVING

½ c brewed coffee

1–2 drops peppermint or mint extract

1 oz dark chocolate or 1 tbsp vegan chocolate chips

⅓ –½ c nondairy milk (plain, chocolate, or vanilla)

Mint leaf and/or crushed vegan chocolate, for garnish (optional)

SINGLE SERVING

1 c nondairy milk

1 tbsp agave nectar

1 tbsp unsweetened cocoa

1 tsp vegan chocolate chips

ground cinnamon

mint mocha

A slimmed down version of the café classic. Skip the hefty price tag (and all the excess sugar, calories, and fat) with this delicious homemade mocha that's perfect during the holidays.

First, brew some ground coffee—one without added flavors works best. Pour ½ cup of the coffee into a mug or thermos. Stir in 1 drop of peppermint or mint extract, followed by the dark chocolate or vegan chocolate chips, stirring until the chocolate melts. Stir in nondairy milk. Taste and add more peppermint if desired. (If you're making this for a guest, you may want to top the mug with a mint leaf and/or crushed chocolate for a more classy presentation.)

hot chocolate

You might remember this recipe from *Happy Herbivore Abroad*. It was so popular that I had to include it in this cookbook. So easy. So delicious.

Combine nondairy milk, agave nectar, cocoa, chocolate chips, and a dash or two ground cinnamon in a blender and whiz until smooth. Gently heat over low in a pan on the stovetop or in the microwave using the beverage setting (or 1–3 minutes, depending on wattage).

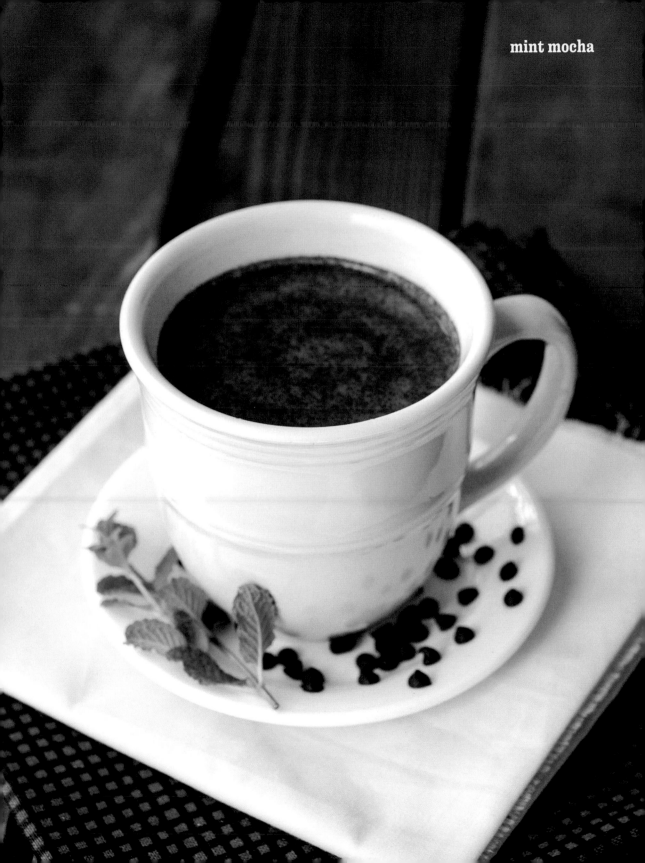

mint mocha

PER SERVING
WITH 1 TBSP MAPLE SYRUP/
WITH 2 TBSP MAPLE SYRUP

Calories 74/126
Fat. 1.3g/1.4g
Carbs 16.0g/29.4g
Fiber 1.6g/1.6g
Sugars. 12g/23.9g
Protein 0.7g/0.7g
WW Points 2

SINGLE SERVING

- 1 c coffee
- ⅓ c unsweetened almond milk (plain or vanilla)
- 1–2 tbsp pure maple syrup or agave nectar
- 1 tsp pumpkin pie spice, plus more if desired for topping
- Pinch ground cinnamon (optional garnish)

pumpkin spice latte

Forget the coffee shop! This sassy little drink is not only vegan (sadly, most pumpkin lattes at coffee shops contain milk products), it has a fraction of the calories and fat of most commercial versions (*and* for a fraction of the price!).

First, brew some ground coffee—one without added flavors works best. Pour 1 cup of the coffee into a mug or thermos. Add almond milk, then stir in 1 tbsp maple syrup and pumpkin pie spice. Taste, adding more maple or spice if desired. If you want to add a bit more sass, top your mug with additional pumpkin pie spice or a pinch of ground cinnamon. For an iced latte, chill your mug (use one large enough to hold additional ice cubes) of pumpkin spice latte in the fridge; then, when you're ready to drink, put several ice cubes into your chilled mug and serve.

pink lemonade

This recipe came to me by way of my friend Chef AJ, who adapted a recipe she learned at a Vitamix demonstration. It's the best pink lemonade I've ever had and it's made strictly from fruit—no sugar!

Zest and juice lemon into a blender. Add frozen and fresh grapes, plus ¼ cup cold water, and blend, adding another ¼ cup water if necessary (add enough water so it blends together). Taste, adding more grapes if it's too tangy.

PER SERVING

Calories	67
Fat	0.3g
Carbs	17.8g
Fiber	0.9g
Sugars	15.5g
Protein	0.7g
WW Points	2

SERVES 2

1 small lemon with zest
1 c frozen red grapes
1 c fresh red grapes

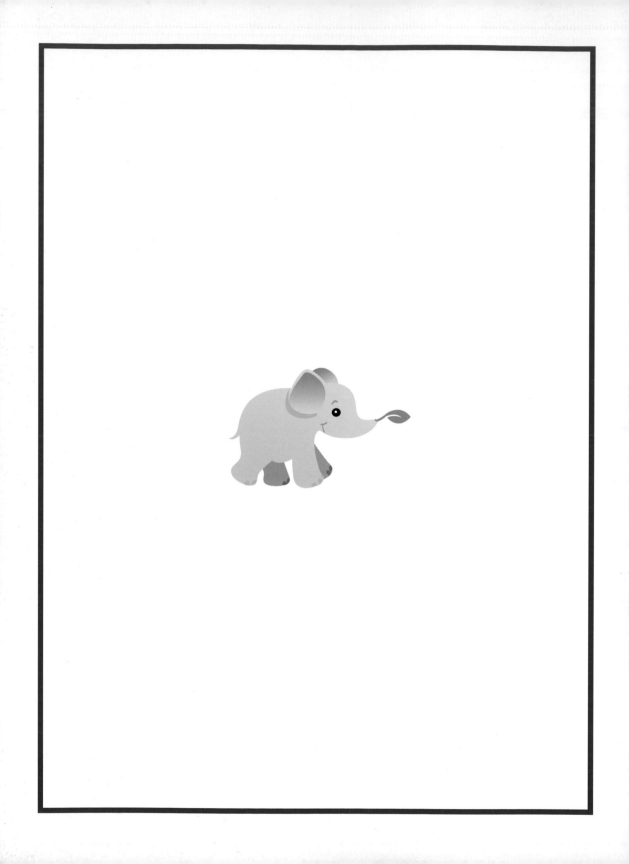

do-it-yourself

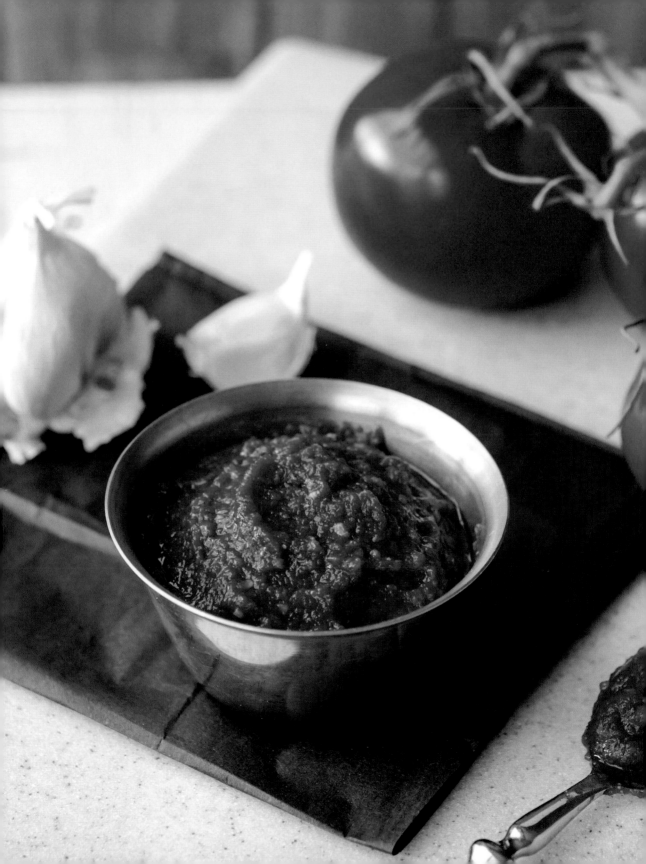

ketchup

I'll be straight with you: Homemade ketchup doesn't exactly taste like Heinz ketchup, but it's delicious in its own right and so much healthier. Less salt, less sugar, no high-fructose corn syrup, and no mystery ingredients! (You'll warm up to homemade ketchup, I promise!)

Whisk all ingredients together, adding more tomato sauce or applesauce as necessary to achieve the right consistency and texture.

Chef's Note I find some vinegars are stronger than others. Start with 1 tbsp, but expect to increase to a total of 1½–2 tbsp. If you like a vinegary ketchup, 2 tbsp should be more than enough. Also, be careful with the allspice—it's potent! A little goes a long way.

PER SERVING
(1 TBSP)

Calories	8
Fat	0g
Carbs	1.8g
Fiber	0g
Sugars	1.2g
Protein	0.3g
WW Points	0

MAKES ½ CUP

1½ tbsp tomato paste

1–2 tbsp apple cider vinegar

2 tbsp unsweetened applesauce

1 tsp onion powder

1 tsp garlic powder

light dash allspice

pinch brown sugar (1 tsp or less)

2 tbsp tomato sauce

salt, to taste

PER 1 TBSP
VEGAN SOUR CREAM (WITH 1 TBSP
AGAVE) / VEGAN MAYO

Calories 13/10
Fat. 0.2g/0.2g
Carbs 1.4g/0.3g
Fiber 0g/0g
Sugars. 1.1g/0g
Protein 1.6g/1.6g
WW Points 0/0

MAKES 1 CUP

- 1 12.3-oz pkg Mori-Nu firm tofu
- 2–4 tbsp lemon juice
- ½ tsp distilled white vinegar
- ⅛ tsp salt
- 1 tsp dry mustard powder
- agave nectar
- granulated garlic powder
- 1 tsp dried or fresh dill (optional)

MAKES 1 CUP

- 1 12.3-oz pkg Mori-Nu tofu
- 2–3 tbsp Dijon mustard
- 2 tsp distilled white vinegar
- lemon juice
- agave nectar

vegan sour cream

This sour cream is easy to make and has a fraction of the fat that dairy and commercial vegan sour creams have.

Combine tofu with 2 tbsp lemon juice, vinegar, salt, mustard powder, a few drops of agave nectar, and a light dash of garlic powder, and blend until smooth and creamy. Taste and add more lemon and/or sweetener if necessary or desired. Stir in dill (if using) before serving.

Chef's Note This sour cream should last at least a week. When tofu goes bad, you know it! It'll turn pink and smell foul.

vegan mayo

Here is my easy and inexpensive recipe for making your own low-fat vegan mayo at home.

Blend tofu with Dijon and vinegar until creamy. Add a few drops of lemon juice and agave nectar, and blend again. Taste and add more lemon, agave nectar, or Dijon as needed. Serve chilled.

marinara sauce

I'm often surprised by how unhealthy commercial pasta sauce is. Almost every jar you pick up contains oil and sugar—neither of which is required to make a good marinara! Several years ago, my best friend Jim turned me on to making my own marinara. It's fast, easy, and so much healthier than store-bought. The little extra effort required is totally worth it, too! Only 35 calories for ¼ cup. Take that, store-bought!

Combine crushed tomatoes and seasonings in a saucepan over medium heat. Bring to a near-boil and reduce heat to medium, continuing to cook for 3 minutes and stirring occasionally. Taste; if too acidic, add agave nectar and more red pepper flakes, if desired. Continue to simmer over low heat for 10–20 minutes, until the herbs lose their raw taste and the sauce is thoroughly warmed.

PER SERVING
(¼ CUP)

Calories 35
Fat. 0.7g
Carbs 5.8g
Fiber 2.1g
Sugars. 4.0g
Protein 1.6g
WW Points 1

MAKES 3 CUPS

- 1 28-oz can crushed tomatoes, with basil
- 2 tbsp Italian seasoning
- ½ tsp granulated garlic powder
- 1 tsp granulated onion powder
- ¼ tsp red pepper flakes, or to taste (optional)
- 1 tsp agave nectar (optional)

PER SERVING
NO-BEEF BROTH (1 CUP) /
NO-CHICKEN BROTH POWDER (1 TBSP)

Calories	27/12
Fat	0.2g/0.1g
Carbs	4.3g/1.7g
Fiber	1.1g/0.7g
Sugars	0.7g/0g
Protein	2.7g/1.3g
WW Points	1/0

MAKES 1 CUP

- 1 tbsp soy sauce or gluten-free tamari
- 1 tbsp nutritional yeast
- ½ tsp Vegan Worcestershire Sauce
- ¼ tsp granulated onion powder
- ¼ tsp granulated garlic powder
- ¼ tsp ground ginger

MAKES ~ 25 SERVINGS

- 1⅓ c nutritional yeast
- 2 tbsp granulated onion powder
- 1 tbsp granulated garlic powder
- 1 tsp dried thyme
- 1 tsp rubbed sage
- 1 tsp paprika
- ½ tsp turmeric
- ¼ tsp celery seed
- ¼ tsp dried parsley

There are a few mock chicken and mock beef broth bouillon cubes on the market, but I find them a little too salty. These are my DIY versions.

no-beef broth

In a medium saucepan, whisk all ingredients together with 1 cup water until well combined. Bring to a boil and simmer for 1 minute.

Chef's Notes

» If you use this broth in a soup recipe, add a bay leaf during cooking.

» If you used low-sodium soy sauce, you might want to add a little salt.

no-chicken broth powder

Combine all ingredients and grind with a mortar and pestle into a fine powder. Store in an airtight container, such as a clear glass jar.

For the broth, mix 1 tablespoon of the mixture with 1 cup warm water to yield 1 cup broth.

vegetable broth

Nothing beats the ease of premade broth or bouillon cubes, but homemade vegetable broth tastes superior in comparison. It's also a great way to use up veggies that are on their way to expiration. I like to use sweet onions, potatoes, parsnips, turnips, and fresh fennel.

Transfer onion, carrot, celery, garlic, and your three additional veggie selections to a large pot. If using dried herbs, grab each green one you have on hand and give it a good shake into the pot. Otherwise, add fresh dill or any complementary fresh herbs you have. Add 1–2 tsp miso, peppercorns, and bay leaf. Add 8 cups cold water, or 10 cups if your vegetable selections are particularly big. Cover and bring to a boil. Reduce heat to low and simmer until the vegetables are falling apart, about one hour. Turn off heat and allow to cool until warm. Use tongs or a spoon to remove bay leaf and vegetables. Grab cheesecloth or a fine strainer and strain liquid into a plastic container. Cool to room temperature, then store in the fridge for up to three days. After three days, store in freezer in 1-cup measurements.

Chef's Note You can omit the miso and add salt to taste for a soy-free vegetable broth.

PER SERVING
(1 CUP)

Calories 49
Fat. 0.4g
Carbs 10.6g
Fiber 2.2g
Sugars. 4.1g
Protein 2.2g
WW Points 1

MAKES 4 CUPS

1 onion (any), peeled
1 large carrot
1 celery stalk
3–4 garlic cloves, peeled

ANY THREE OF THE FOLLOWING:

1 small brown potato
2–4 small red potatoes
1 c mushrooms
1 bell pepper, seeded
1 medium turnip
1 medium zucchini
1 parsnip
3–5 oz fresh or dried herbs (any)
1–2 tsp yellow miso
4 whole black peppercorns
1 bay leaf

PER SERVING
(1 TSP)

Calories 6
Fat. 0g
Carbs 0.9g
Fiber 0g
Sugars. 0.6g
Protein 0.3g
WW Points 0

MAKES 1 CUP

- 6 tbsp apple cider vinegar
- 2 tbsp tamari
- 1 tbsp brown sugar or 1 tsp molasses
- 2 tsp prepared mustard (any)
- ¼ tsp granulated onion powder
- ¼ tsp granulated garlic powder
- ¼ tsp ground ginger
- ⅛ tsp ground cinnamon
- cayenne pepper or chili powder
- allspice or ground cloves

Chef's Note Yeast extract, such as Marmite or Vegemite, can be used in place of Worcestershire sauce if Worcestershire sauce is being used as an ingredient in something and not as a condiment or marinade.

vegan worcestershire sauce

Most commercial Worcestershire sauces contain anchovies, although there are a few vegetarian brands on the market. While nothing beats the ease of bottled sauce, this DIY recipe is allergen-free and very inexpensive to make. Worcestershire sauce is traditionally used as a condiment for meat, and consequently is a great marinade for veggie burgers and acts as a flavoring agent in many meat-substitute recipes.

Whisk all ingredients from vinegar through ground cinnamon together and add a light dash of cayenne or chili powder and a light dash of allspice or ground cloves with ¼ cup water until well combined. Add salt, if desired. Store in an airtight container in the fridge.

brody's gluten-free flour blend

Brody's Bakery (brodysbakcry.com) is Kansas City's only all-vegan and gluten-free bakery. This is their tried-and-true recipe for gluten-free all-purpose flour and it's used in all of their scrumptious goodies. "We've burned through a lot of gluten-free flour blends and this seems to be the only one that (a) no one can tell is gluten-free, and (b) works with any recipe, be it for cooking or baking," says Katie Olson, owner and baker.

Mix all ingredients together. Store in an airtight container and use cup for cup anytime whole-wheat or all-purpose flour is called for in a recipe.

PER ¼ CUP

Calories 46
Fat. 0.6g
Carbs 33.5g
Fiber 1g
Sugars. 0g
Protein 1.4g
WW Points 4

MAKES 2 CUPS

TO REPLACE 2 C OF FLOUR

1 c brown rice flour
½ c tapioca starch
½ c potato starch

plus 1 tsp xanthan gum or guar gum for every 2 c of this blend

PER SERVING
POULTRY SEASONING MIX (1 TBSP) /
BAKED POTATOES (PER POTATO)

Calories	10/131
Fat	0.4g/0.1g
Carbs	2.0g/29.7g
Fiber	1.3g/3.7g
Sugars	0g/1.3g
Protein	0.3g/3.4g
WW Points	0/3

MAKES ¼ CUP

- 1 tbsp dried rosemary
- 1 tbsp dried thyme
- 1 tbsp rubbed sage (not powdered)
- 1 tbsp dried marjoram or oregano
- 1 tbsp dried parsley or basil

Chef's Note If you can find granulated (not powdered) poultry seasoning that isn't a rub, feel free to use it for convenience instead of blending your own. I like Cost Plus World Market's generic brand.

YIELD AMOUNT VARIES

- potatoes
- foil

poultry seasoning mix

This savory herb mixture is my favorite seasoning. You can substitute store-bought poultry blends for convenience; just be sure they're not powdered. The consistency should be like dried basil. In a pinch, Italian seasoning may be substituted.

Grind herbs together in a mortar and pestle until coarse like the consistency of sea salt, but not powdered. Store in an airtight container.

slow-cooked baked potatoes

This isn't so much a recipe as a tip from my friend Kim. (I know, I know, I'm weird for not owning a slow cooker, but I just don't have the patience to wait 8 hours when I can make something in 8 minutes!)

Wash your potatoes well and let them dry. Wrap in foil (do not prick skin). Place in a dry slow cooker (e.g., Crock-Pot) and cook on low for 6 hours. Ta-da! Baked potatoes when you get home from work.

hummus

Cedar's makes a totally fat-free (oil-free) hummus available exclusively at Whole Foods Market. Many supermarkets are now selling lower-fat hummus varieties, but they may still contain oil. Here's my basic oil-free and no-added-fat hummus recipe, meaning it does not contain tahini (a sesame seed paste).

In a blender or food processor, combine chickpeas, lemon juice, ground cumin, ground coriander, garlic powder, Dijon, and miso (if using). Allow the motor to run until the beans are chopped up. Stop, scrape the sides, and add 1 tbsp broth. Allow the motor to run again, adding more broth as necessary, until the mixture achieves a smooth, hummus consistency. (I typically use 3 ½ tbsp broth.) You may need to stop and scrape the sides periodically. Once consistency is achieved, taste, adding more lemon or Dijon if desired (a little goes a long way!).

PER SERVING
(1 TBSP)

Calories 21
Fat 0.2g
Carbs 3.3g
Fiber 0.8g
Sugars 0g
Protein 1.1g
WW Points 0

MAKES ABOUT 1 CUP

1 15-oz can chickpeas, drained and rinsed

juice of ½ small lemon

½ tsp ground cumin

½ tsp ground coriander

¼ tsp granulated garlic powder

1 tsp Dijon mustard

¼ tsp yellow miso (white or red miso work too; optional)

vegetable broth, as needed

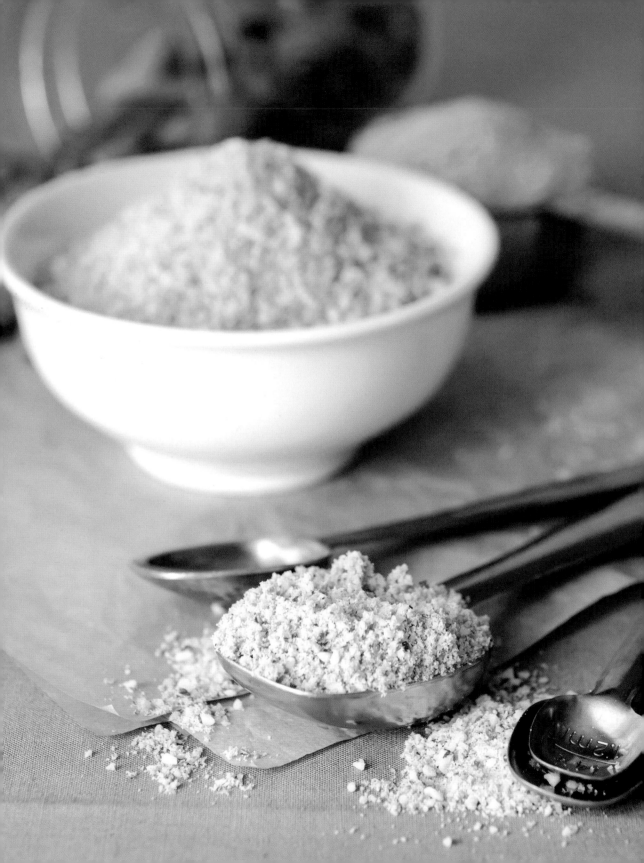

aj's vegan parmesan

There are two commercial brands of vegan Parmesan cheese on the market: Galaxy Global and Parma. If you can't find these where you live (or you want a slightly less processed DIY option), here is a great alternative recipe by my friend Chef AJ.

AJ says, "I put one cup of nuts and half a cup of nutritional yeast in the blender. I add one tbsp of salt-free seasoning, but you could use a little salt or even garlic powder and/or onion powder. But even just the nuts and 'nooch' [nutritional yeast] are good. I use whatever nuts I have on hand, which could be raw almonds, raw cashews, or even raw Brazil nuts. It's also really good with ½ cup raw walnuts and ½ cup raw sunflower seeds!" Process until a smooth powder has formed. Store in an airtight container in the fridge for a week.

PER SERVING
(1 TBSP, WITH CASHEWS)

Calories	45
Fat	2.8g
Carbs	3.4g
Fiber	1g
Sugars	0g
Protein	2.4g
WW Points	1

MAKES 1½ CUPS

1 c nuts
½ c nutritional yeast
pinch salt or salt-free seasoning

Chef's Note I've also seen recipes online using sesame seeds. I imagine any of these options, or even a combination, would be great. You can also start with less nutritional yeast (3–4 tbsp), adding more to taste.

THE NUMBERS GAME: MY BATTLE WITH THE SCALE

After years of running around in high heels and carrying a heavy laptop on my shoulder (and before that, while in school, heavy books), I developed a number of muscle imbalances and other musculoskeletal problems. Because I was slender and otherwise felt good (except for occasional stiffness and muscle pain), I was unaware that I had any physical problems—I thought I was fine. However, I knew sitting at my desk all day working wasn't exactly good for my body, so I started doing yoga to combat my workday immobility.

I realized rather quickly that I wasn't exactly what you'd call limber, but my agility and flexibility improved week by week. Fast forward to a few months later. I treated myself to a deep-tissue massage and afterward my massage therapist asked if I carried a heavy handbag or laptop all the time, noting my muscles were very unbalanced.

This surprised and concerned me, so I made an appointment with a physical therapist who was also a personal trainer. My initial evaluation was embarrassing. Even I could tell just how bad it was. My hips and shoulders were pronated. I was walking incorrectly. My calves and hamstrings were tight. My right side was exponentially stronger than my left (muscle imbalances all around) and my posture left much to be desired (that I knew before the consultation!).

We started working together immediately to correct my problems. As part of my "therapy," I was required to complete a number of exercises with weights or just using my body weight (push-ups, for example). After several weeks on the program, I could tell I was getting stronger. I could see and feel the difference in my body—I was now "fixing" it.

Now, there is a point to all this! I thought that with all my new "exercise," I might have shed a little weight and so I decided to hop on the scale for an ego boost. Instead I was shocked. I'd *gained* six pounds since starting my program. At first I panicked. I thought, "How could I gain weight? I've been eating so well!" And I had been. It was so disheartening. For two years I'd maintained my weight without exercising by following a low-fat, plant-based diet, and now that I'd become a bit more active I gained weight! Something was wrong with this picture.

That's when I checked my body fat percentage. It had gone down. My weight had increased because I'd put on muscle—muscle that I needed to correct all my problems! It was a reminder to me that numbers on a scale are not necessarily a true or absolute indicator of health. The scale is a helpful tool, yes, but weight is just a piece of the whole puzzle. Just because I weighed six pounds more than I did two months earlier didn't mean I was less healthy. I was actually *healthier* because I had started fixing my body and improving my strength. Meanwhile, my clothes were fitting better and I'd received some warm compliments from friends and coworkers—much more valuable than numbers on a scale!

> **Numbers on a scale are not necessarily a true or absolute indicator of health.**

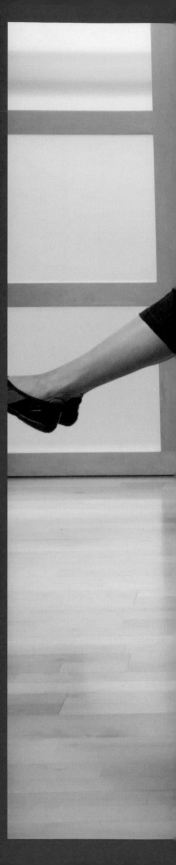

LEAN

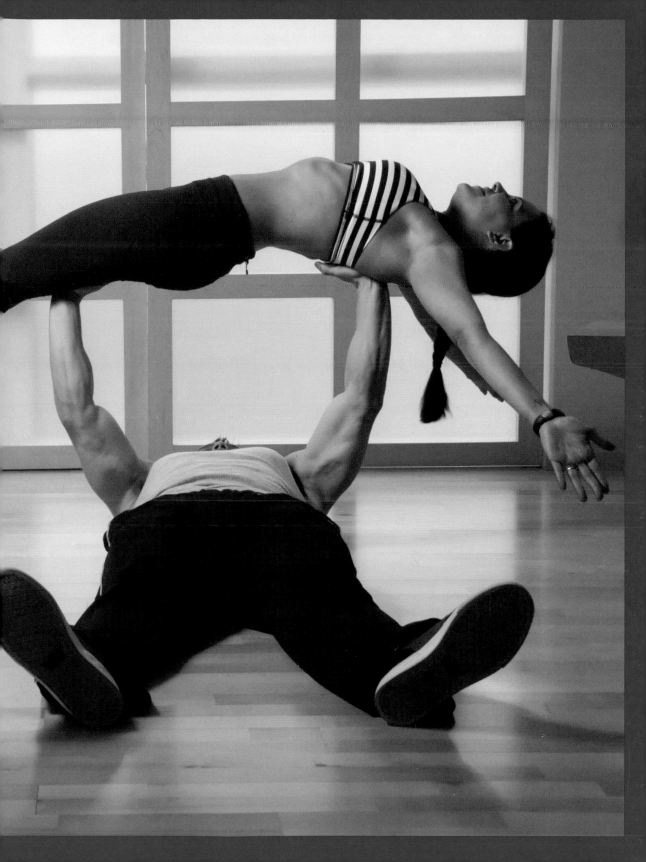

is exercise required?

Is exercise *required* to lose weight? Absolutely not. I've worked with dozens of people who lost weight without exercise by simply changing their diets.

My family is a great testimonial to this. My parents don't exercise beyond the normal walking required to live their lives, and within a few months of changing to a low-fat, whole-foods, plant-based diet, they lost a whopping 40 pounds together. My sister, meanwhile, moved closer to me last year and started coming over to my house for the majority of her meals. Other than walking eight minutes between my house and hers, she was not exercising, and within six months she lost more than 20 pounds—something she had not been able to do schlepping to the gym for an hour several days a week. Neither my parents nor my sister had set out to lose weight; the shedding of pounds was merely an added bonus to their dietary changes.

THE BENEFITS OF EXERCISE

So that begs the question: Why bother to exercise?

While many of us turn to exercise for vanity or weight loss (or a combination), exercise is also a key part of a healthy lifestyle beyond how it makes our pants fit. Regular exercise improves our mood, helps combat stress, eases anxiety and depression, boosts self-confidence, helps prevent injury, and keeps our body functioning properly.

Another great reason is that adding exercise into your lifestyle can help expedite weight loss by torching calories (see the 100 Factor—Fitness [pg. 278]), and when you put on muscle from exercise, you'll burn even more calories when you're not working out, which leads to even more weight loss. This is because an increase in muscle mass boosts your RMR (resting metabolic rate)—the rate at which your body burns calories. Even when we're sleeping, we're still burning calories.

However, quicker weight loss is not the only reason I champion exercise. I'm in it for the benefits beyond the scale. I first started exercising to lose weight and then continued to exercise out of fear I'd gain back all the weight I had lost. When I stopped exercising, yet maintained my weight, I decided to return to exercising so I could fix muscular imbalances in my body.

Exercise definitely helped my strength and flexibility, but I found other benefits, too. The obvious was I became more self-confident. I also noticed that my mood improved. I wasn't just happier; my moods were also more stable and consistent.

Before long, I started scheduling exercise in my day planner under the guise of "therapy" because these times often became self-therapy sessions as well: my time alone with my thoughts and feelings. Interestingly, I also found that solutions to problems that had been plaguing me came to me while I was exercising. One time, I distinctly remember leaving work in a fit of frustration over a problem I couldn't solve. I went for a run to "clear my head" and to de-stress. Twenty-five minutes later, at around mile three, the solution to the problem bubbled up in my thoughts. Some of my best ideas come to me while I am exercising.

> **I'm a better person when I exercise regularly; it's that simple.**

If you do an online search for "exercise benefits," you'll find all the perks I experience are par for the course. I'm a better person when I exercise regularly; it's that simple. Plus, you just feel awesome when you're all sweaty and pooped after a workout! Remember, even if you take it slow and modify, you're still showing up anyone on the couch! We all start somewhere, even me—as I mentioned in the introduction to this book, it wasn't that long ago that I was too out of shape to walk a 5K for charity!

Exercise is not required for weight loss, but I find I'm my best self when I exercise regularly—and I want you to be *your* best self too! Let's be our best selves together! Let's be light *and* lean.

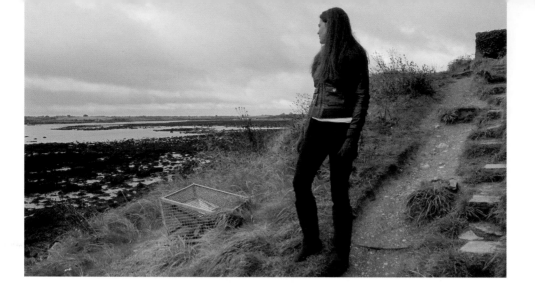

the 100 factor—fitness

Remember the 100 Factor—Calories concept from earlier in this cookbook? Here's the short version: If you torch 100 extra calories a day, you can lose *10 pounds* by the end of the year. No trip to the gym required!

Here are 42 easy ways to burn off 100 calories in your day-to-day life.* Some take as little as 10 minutes! *Feel the burn.* Go do one right now!

P. S. If you cook for 34 minutes, you burn 100 calories. What a motivation to eat in!

Based on a 150-pound individual.

I've had a lot of questions from readers who are not losing weight despite eating a plant-based diet. I discuss multiple factors to consider here: http://herbi.es/WhyNoWeightLoss.

30 MINUTES OR LESS

1. Bowling–30 minutes
2. Driving Range/Mini Golf–30 minutes
3. Frisbee–30 minutes
4. House Cleaning (moderate)–25 minutes
5. Ironing 25 minutes
6. Walking the Dog–25 minutes
7. Carrying an Infant–24 minutes
8. Pilates–24 minutes
9. Bike Riding (casually)–23 minutes
10. Raking Leaves–23 minutes
11. Playing with Kids–23 minutes
12. Sweeping–23 minutes
13. Vacuuming–23 minutes

20 MINUTES OR LESS

14. Basketball–20 minutes
15. House Work (vigorous)–20 minutes
16. Mopping–20 minutes
17. Mowing the Lawn–20 minutes
18. Walking (3 mph)–20 minutes
19. Washing Car–20 minutes
20. Yoga–20 minutes
21. Ice Skating (moderate)–18 minutes
22. Painting House–18 minutes
23. Softball/Baseball–18 minutes
24. Weeding–18 minutes

15 MINUTES OR LESS

25. Dancing–15 minutes
26. Gardening–15 minutes
27. Golfing (carrying clubs)–15 minutes
28. Lifting Weights (vigorously)–15 minutes
29. Shoveling Snow–15 minutes
30. Swimming (moderate intensity)–15 minutes
31. Tennis (single)–15 minutes
32. Walking (briskly)–15 minutes
33. Water Skiing–15 minutes
34. Kickball–13 minutes
35. Soccer (casual)–13 minutes
36. Jog in Place–12 minutes
37. Zumba–11 minutes

10 MINUTES OR LESS

38. Skiing (downhill)–10 minutes
39. Jumping Rope (moderate intensity)–9 minutes
40. Running (6 mph)–9 minutes
41. Elliptical–8 minutes
42. Running Stairs–6 minutes

MAKING EXERCISE HAPPEN

Through being a personal trainer as well as through my own workout sessions, I've learned that crafting a lifestyle with time for fitness built into it isn't easy—unless you plan. Here are a few tricks for making regular workouts a reality and not just a lofty aspiration!

#1 Schedule it. Whether you write it on your to-do list, create an appointment on your calendar, or write it on your hand, schedule a workout. Treat fitness time like you'd treat any other important meeting or event (say, a conference call with the boss or a friend's birthday bash). My motto is "I don't find time for fitness; I make time."

#2 Lay it all out. Before you go to bed, lay out all your gym clothes on a chair in your bedroom, complete with your socks, sneakers, water bottle, and anything else you might need. You'll be less likely to hit the snooze button with those clothes staring at you—*and* you'll have to walk right by them before leaving the bedroom. I find taking that first step also helps solidify my commitment to my workout the next day. If you exercise after work, pack your gym bag and leave it by the front door so you take it with you to work. Don't leave it in your car! Keep it in your office so you have to take it with you when you leave—you won't forget about your commitment on your way home. It's in your hand along with your keys, reminding you!

#3 Make a date. Every Sunday at 9 A.M.—rain or shine—I go for a hike with my friend Blyth. While I can easily persuade myself to stay in bed a little later on a gloomy day, I can't bring myself to let Blyth down. We keep each other in check. Social commitments rule!

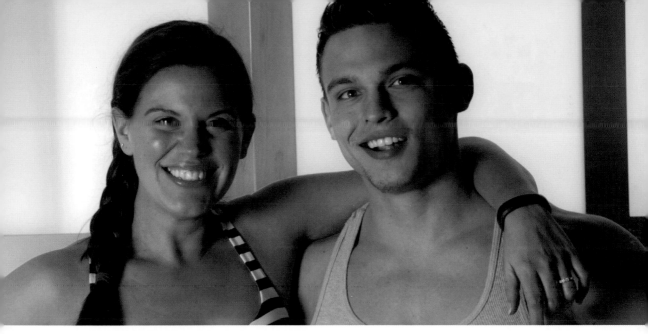

fitness workouts

I've teamed up with my friend Jon Warren—a certified personal trainer and physical therapy aide—to create easy, no-fuss exercises. Whether you're a beginner or an advanced thrill-seeker, these workouts (or "body recipes" as I like to call them) will help keep you lean and healthy.*

Jon is originally from Houston, Texas, and graduated with a degree in finance from Texas Tech University. He works as a certified personal trainer and physical therapy aide in Orange County, California, where he runs the training department for the largest Gold's Gym in the state. He holds National Academy of Sports Medicine (NASM) and National Council for Certified Personal Trainers (NCCPT) certifications and is certified with kettlebells and in TRX Suspension Training. Jon also serves as a corrective exercise specialist and performance enhancement specialist through NASM. He is currently a National Physique Committee (NPC) Men's Physique competitor.

Now. . . let's get fit!

Please consult your doctor before beginning any exercise program.

let's work out!

HOW IT WORKS: Do two or three sets of each move with a 30-second rest between each, or if you're just starting out, run through it all once and repeat if you can. (Beginners: Take breaks as you need them!) Perform this workout two or three times per week. If possible, slip in 20 to 60 minutes of cardio—swimming, riding your bike, going for a walk, dancing in your living room—one or two days a week to go along with it. Make it a social event and invite your friends!

1. BASIC FRONT LUNGE

Start by standing upright. Step one foot forward, allowing both knees to bend so the thigh on the forward leg is parallel to the floor and the knee of the rear leg is about 1 inch above the floor. Push off the front foot to stand back up in the starting position. (Make sure your front knee does not go over your front foot or ankle). Alternate legs for 15 reps each.

MODIFIED: Do five reps for each leg (you could also do a back lunge instead; it's much easier).

HARDER: Increase reps and/or add weights in your hands (e.g., 10 pounds).

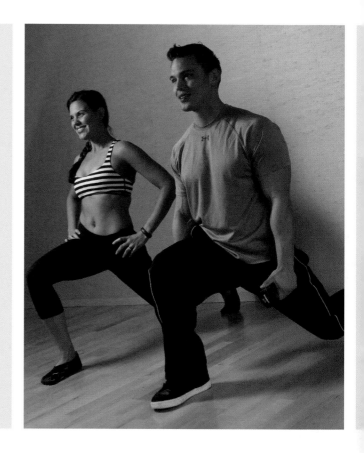

2. ASSISTED PUSH-UP

Start on your knees, putting a towel under them for comfort if necessary. Lean forward slightly (keeping your back straight) and place your palms on the floor, shoulder width apart. Keep your feet together and off the floor. (Your body looks like it's the shape of an N.) Bend your elbows, lowering your body to the floor. (Keep your abs engaged and your back straight—do not arch your back.) Once your nose is an inch from the floor, push upward, straightening your arms (but don't lock your elbows) and moving your body back into the starting position. Repeat 10 to 15 times.

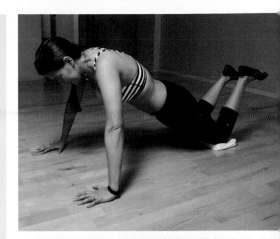

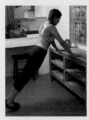

MODIFIED: Wall Push-Ups: Stand in front of a bare wall with your arms extended out straight in front of you. Place your palms on the wall, shoulder width apart (your fingertips pointing to the ceiling). Back your feet up a few steps (the farther away from the wall, the more challenging it is); your elbows should bend as you lean toward the wall at an incline. Keeping your back straight (do not arch your back) and while engaging your abs, lower your body toward the wall and then push yourself back up for one rep.

HARDER: Full military-style push-ups, on your hands and toes (knees up!). You can make it slightly easier by separating your feet by a few inches. Need it even harder? Try doing military push-ups with one leg in the air!

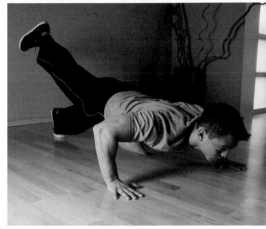

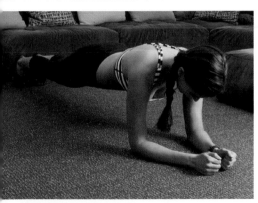

3. PLANK

Start in the military push-up position. Go down on your elbows, so that you're resting your weight on your forearms. You can clasp your hands together (keeping your hands apart makes it harder). Keep your back and body straight as a board with your abs engaged. Don't arch your back or let your hips fall toward the ground. Hold the position for 30 seconds, or as long as you can.

MODIFIED: Take three-second breaks as necessary by dropping your knees down to rest briefly.

HARDER: Do not clasp hands. Hold for as long as possible—two minutes = super warrior! Another option is to do a side plank. Start off this static contraction exercise by lying on your right side, propping yourself up with your right forearm and elbow planted at your side. Your left arm is extended, resting on your left thigh. Your right hip and leg should be touching the floor. Begin by raising your hips until your body forms a straight line from head to ankle, keeping the side of your right foot on the floor with the left foot stacked on top. Your points of contact to the floor will be your elbow and forearm and the side of your foot and ankle. Hold this for 15 to 60 seconds.

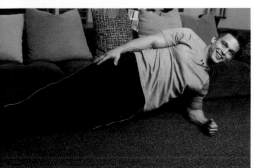

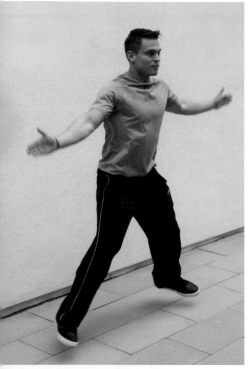

4. JUMPING JACKS

Start in the standing position with your arms by your sides. Jump your feet apart and while you do this, bring your arms up in a semicircular motion, with your hands over your head. After you land, jump your legs back together while bringing your arms back down in a semicircular motion. Repeat for 30 seconds or 50 jacks.

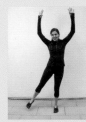

MODIFIED: Low-Impact Jumping Jacks: Instead of jumping out with both legs at the same time, extend just one leg out at a time as you bring your hands together. When you lower your arms, step together and then alternate to the other leg as you raise them again. Shoot for 20 repetitions.

HARDER: Jumping Jacks with Toe Touch: Start like a normal jumping jack, but as you finish the motion, bend both knees and perform a squat, touching your toes. Spring right back into a jumping jack and repeat 20 to 60 times.

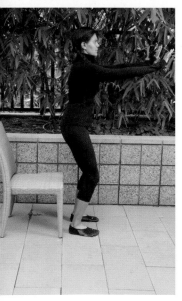

5. BODY SQUAT

Stand in front of a chair with your feet shoulder width apart. With your arms out in front of you and the weight on your heels (not your toes), lower yourself down as if you're about to sit down on the chair. As soon as your bottom skims the top of the chair, rise back up to standing position. I find doing this exercise barefoot and lifting my toes (make sure your knees don't come out over the toes) helps ensure I have proper form.

MODIFIED: Squat into a chair, rest, repeat.

HARDER: Hold weight (e.g., 10-pound dumbbells) on your shoulders.

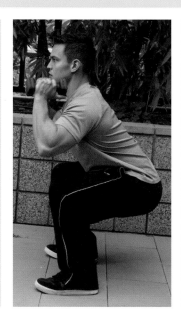

6. DIPS

Sit on a bench with your legs straight out in front of you, feet resting flat on the floor. While holding onto the bench (your arms straight and close to your sides, palms connected with the bench, fingers facing forward and hugging under the bench), slide yourself forward so your bottom is off the bench. Lower yourself until your bottom almost touches the ground (your arms should make 90-degree angles here), then push yourself back up into the starting position. For best results, keep the up and down movements controlled and even. Do 15 reps.

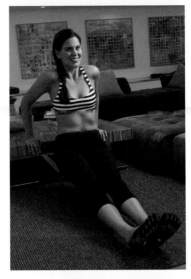

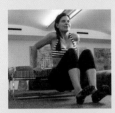

MODIFIED: Place your feet flat on the floor, your legs making a 90-degree angle from your seat on the bench. For a slightly harder approach, stay on your heels, not your entire foot.

HARDER: Place your feet up on a chair or bench across from you and dip. You can also add weight to your lap.

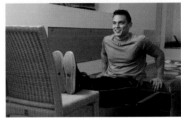

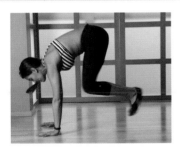

7. BURPEES

Begin in a standing position. Drop into a squat position, placing your palms on the ground next to your feet (outside your feet). Thrust your legs backward into a front plank ("push-up") position. Jump your legs back up to your hands and return to a standing position.

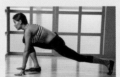

MODIFIED: Walk your legs back and forward from standing position to front plank back to standing.

HARDER: Add a push-up in the plank position and hop straight up and down once you've returned to the standing position. Still not tough enough? Perform this exercise on one leg!

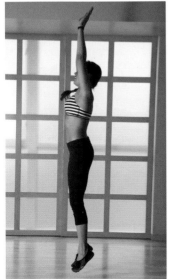

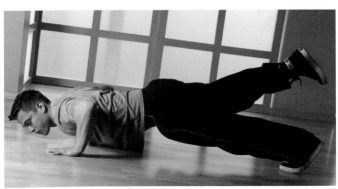

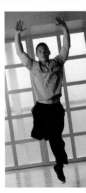

8. PLIÉ SQUATS

Stand with your legs 2 to 3 feet apart with toes turned out like a ballerina. With your hands on your hips, push hips back and lower your body until your thighs are parallel to the floor. Pause, then push back up into starting position. That's one rep. Repeat 15 times.

MODIFIED: Place a chair in front of you and use it for support.

HARDER: Add weights (e.g., 10-pound dumbbells). Rest weights on your thigh, but hold them with your hands.

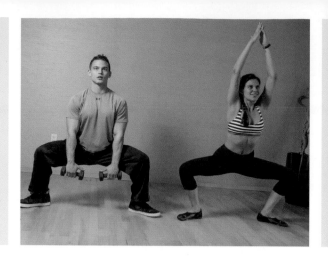

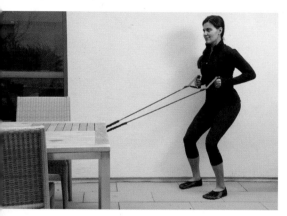

9. STANDING ROWS

Wrap a resistance band around a fixed object such as a pole that allows you to pull the handles to your mid-torso. Take a step or two back and slightly bend your knees. Holding the handles lightly, extend your arms forward fully. Your chest should be high and your shoulders back (think of someone putting a coat on you). Squeeze your shoulder blades together. With your palms facing each other, pull the band back toward your midsection. Keep your elbows tight to your sides, squeezing your shoulder blades together even tighter. Slowly return to starting position and repeat.

MODIFIED: The farther away you are from the fixed object, the more resistance you will experience. There are also different levels of bands (some are easier than others). You can also squat down more and fire up the glutes, hamstrings, and quads.

HARDER: Stand upright (keep your back straight) with weights (e.g., dumbbells, cans, or even a phone book) in your hands—just resting in front of you, not holding away from the body. Pull your arms upward so your elbows rise toward the ceiling and the weights are at your chest, below your chin. The weights should be close to the body as you move them upward. Now slowly lower the weights back down. Repeat 15 times. Still not hard enough? Use heavier weights!

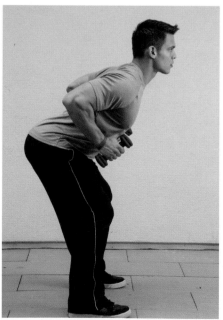

10. KNEELING ARM AND LEG REACH

On a mat or cushy towel, get on your hands and knees. (Your arms should be under your shoulders and your knees under your hips.) Face the ground. Keep your back straight like a tabletop, engaging your abs. Reach your left arm straight out in front of you while lifting your right leg out straight behind you, tightening your glutes. Bring both back in, trying to touch your elbow to the opposite knee under your abdomen. Repeat five to fifteen times. Then switch to your other arm and leg.

MODIFIED: Extend your opposite arm and leg the same way, but don't try to bring your elbow to your knee. Alternate sides after each rep.

HARDER: Perform the modified movement from your hands and toes.

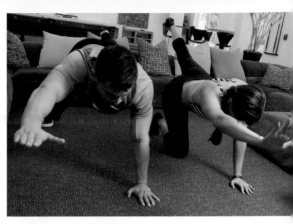

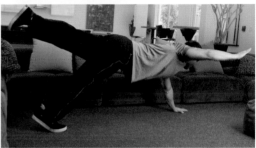

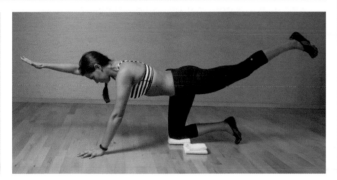

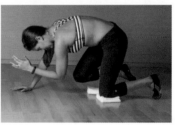

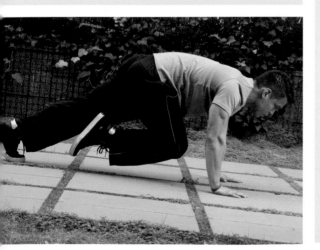

11. MOUNTAIN CLIMBERS

Start in a push-up position, with your palms on the ground and your shoulders directly over your hands. Pull your right knee toward your chest, toe on the ground, then thrust your leg back out behind you, with your toe on the ground. As you thrust your right leg back, pull your left knee toward your chest (toe on the ground), then kick the left leg back out as the right knee and toe come in. Alternate legs, doing this motion as fast as possible for 30 seconds.

MODIFIED: Elevate your torso by placing your hands on a bench, table, or chair, rather than on the ground.

HARDER: Continue the motion for as long as possible, at least 45 seconds.

lindsay's body blast

This all-in-one exercise is what I do when my time (and space) is limited. It's a little on the *advanced* side, so you may need to work up to it. It's a killer circuit and I have a lot of fun challenging myself, drill-instructor style, to see how fast I can move through the exercise (while still keeping proper form!) and how many rounds I can go through before I'm wasted. (Usually two, but I'm a work in progress!)

Start by standing upright with your arms out straight ahead. Sit back into a squat (keep the weight on your heels) and then place palms on the floor, next to your feet. Thrust legs back into a plank position. Tighten abs, keep back straight, and bring your left knee to the inside of your right arm, then extend back to starting position. Bring your right knee to the inside of your left arm, then extend back to starting position. Bring your right knee to the outside of your right elbow, then extend back to starting position. Bring your left knee to the outside of your left elbow, then extend back to starting position.

With toes on the floor (dropping to knees if necessary) do a push-up. Roll over on to your back. Keeping your head, shoulders, and feet on the floor, thrust your hips up into an angled bridge. Repeat five times, really squeezing the glutes. Next, place hands on the floor near your ears, finger tips pointing back at your shoulders, feet planted, and lift your body up into a full wheel (or table-top) and hold for as long as you can. Slowly lower yourself back down. Do a few crunches or sit-ups, then lift your legs straight in the air, perpendicular to the floor. Tighten your abs and lift your butt and hips off the ground so your legs go straight up toward the sky. Lower back down and repeat a few times. Lower your legs to the ground and roll your body back up into the standing position. Repeat the circuit.

testimonials

Many people have shaved off pounds by changing to a low-fat, whole foods, plant-based diet. You can find dozens of stories attesting to this at Getmealplans.com and as part of the herbie of the week series on happyherbivore.com, http://herbi.es/Herbies. As you'll read, most of the success stories do not involve exercise, just a new approach to eating—the Happy Herbivore way! The following testimonials come from meal plan and Happy Herbivore cookbook users. You'll find even more like this in the Amazon.com reviews for my cookbooks. *Changing your diet changes everything and it is enough on its own to achieve weight loss and to maintain that loss while looking and feeling fabulous!*

I am just so happy on your plan. It is amazing. I started two weeks ago. This morning I weighed myself and I have lost six pounds!! This is with no other changes, no exercise and while eating an enormous amount of delicious food. *(Update: "11 months later, I have now lost 45 lbs!")*

—LINDA W.

In three months I have lost 42 pounds! I'm only 5'2", so that weight loss has been significant! I do not exercise, except for what I get walking around at work. I use your individual meal plans."

—P. G.

"I have lost 50 pounds since going vegan and I have your cookbooks to thank for that! I went from 280 to 230 [pounds] without exercise and I am still going! It has changed my life forever!"

—APRIL GARDNER

"We cook from your books and use your meal plan recipes. We eat Happy Herbivore recipes around 75% of the time. I've lost 15 pounds and my fiancé has lost 7 pounds. Neither of us exercises."

—J. B.

"I started cooking from the Happy Herbivore cookbooks and was amazed at how fast and easy and delicious the recipes were! But the best part? I've been steadily losing weight—without exercising! I am definitely sticking with this—it works for me!"

—JENNIE F.

"Your meal plans and cookbooks have totally changed my life. In a few months time I have lost 35 pounds. I went from a size 14 to a size 4 without exercise. I also no longer take any meds, my acid reflux and digestive problems are gone, and my cholesterol went from 259 to 140 [mg/dL]. I am a new woman and I have never felt better."

—MARSHA O.

"I lost 45 pounds by using your cookbooks. I have a bad back and am generally lazy, so with the exception of doggie walks I didn't really exercise."

—CAROLYN LEONARD

"Trying to kick the last 10 pounds post-baby, I faithfully did a workout DVD every day for a month. Discouraged with no change to my weight, I quit. Several months later I started following the Happy Herbivore [diet]—cut out meat, dairy, and oil, and used many of Lindsay's recipes. Within a few months, the 10 pounds were gone—just from changing the way I ate."

—LISA M.

"After my second child, I struggled to lose weight. It took me four months to lose 10 pounds on WW [Weight Watchers], but [I] lost the remaining 20 in about two months using Happy Herbivore recipes! Without exercise!"

—SARAH B.

"All I did to lose 16 pounds was follow the recipes in your book; it was that simple. I look forward to losing more weight."

—CORY T.

"I lost 17 pounds without doing anything other than sticking to eating delicious recipes from the Happy Herbivore cookbooks. I consistently lost a pound every week, and that was without exercising. I've kept that weight off, too."

—SARA M.

"In the past year, neither my husband nor I have done much exercise other than taking the occasional walk, and yet we have both enjoyed significant weight loss. I have lost 58 pounds and my husband has lost about 45. We cook multiple Happy Herbivore recipes a week."

—MICHELLE M.

"We use your cookbooks and meal plans. Without exercise, I have lost 30 pounds and was able to wear a smaller dress at my recent wedding. I work in an office at a desk all day and I never dreamed weight loss would be so easy."

—AMANDA G.

"I turned to a plant-based diet in hopes of losing 10 pounds. That was 20 months ago, and in that time I have lost 50 pounds!! I lost that weight simply by changing what I ate, and not through exercise. I cook almost exclusively from Happy Herbivore."

—CATHY H.

"It's been two-and-a-half weeks cooking your recipes, and with NO change in exercise or anything else, my husband has lost 17 pounds!"

—E. F.

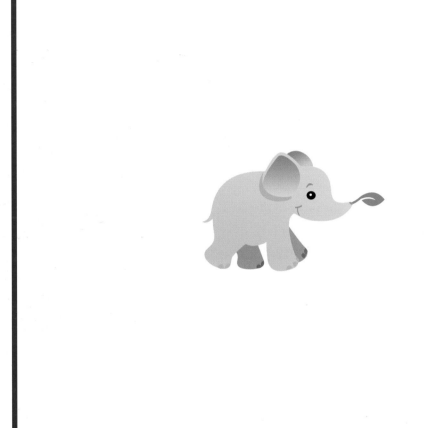

appendix

glossary of ingredients

AGAVE NECTAR

Pronounced ah-GAH-vay, agave nectar is a natural, unrefined sweetener with a consistency similar to honey. It comes from the agave plant, which also is used to make tequila. It can replace honey, sugar, and maple syrup in recipes and works especially well as a sweetener in drinks.

APPLE CIDER VINEGAR

This very acidic and strong-smelling vinegar is made from apples or cider. It is often combined with nondairy milk to sour it into vegan buttermilk. It's also used for flavor and served instead of ketchup with sweet potato fries. Apple cider vinegar can be found in most grocery stores, but you can substitute lemon juice if necessary.

BLACK SALT

Black salt is also called *kala namak*. Not to be confused with Hawaiian black lava salt.

BROTHS

Use any light-colored vegetable broth from bouillon or homemade broth. When possible, buy no-salt-added or low-sodium options.

BROWN RICE

Bran and germ—key nutrients in rice—have been removed to make white rice white, but brown rice is what white rice once was. To save time, stock up on precooked brown rice that reheats in about a minute.

COCOA

Most unsweetened cocoa powders are unintentionally vegan. Hershey's and Ghirardelli are good brands to try.

COLLARD GREENS

These leafy greens are an excellent source of fiber and vitamin C. Find them at health food stores and most well-stocked supermarkets. When preparing the greens, be sure to remove the ribs by running a sharp knife along each side.

CONFECTIONERS' SUGAR
See powdered sugar.

COOKING SPRAY
An aerosol designated as a high-heat cooking spray or an oil spray can filled with high-heat cooking oil.

GRANULATED ONION AND GARLIC POWDERS
Look for onion and garlic powders that are granulated, resembling the consistency of fine salt, and not powders that are similar to flour or confectioners' sugar (the latter are sometimes called California-style spices).

INDIAN SPICES
Indian spices such as turmeric, coriander, garam masala, ground cumin, curry powder, and fennel seeds can be found in most health food stores but are very inexpensive at Indian stores and online.

ITALIAN SEASONING
Italian seasoning is a blend of basil, rosemary, thyme, sage, marjoram, and oregano. In a pinch, Poultry Seasoning Mix (pg. 268) can be substituted.

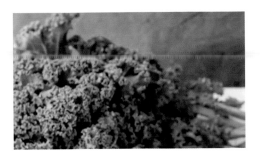

KALE
This leafy green is an excellent source of antioxidants, beta carotene, vitamins K and C, and calcium. Kale can be found at health food stores and most well-stocked supermarkets. I prefer the dark, deep green Lacinato kale commonly labeled dinosaur kale. When preparing kale, be sure to remove the ribs by running a sharp knife along each side.

LIQUID SMOKE
Found in most supermarkets, liquid smoke is smoke condensation captured in water. It looks like low-sodium soy sauce but smells like barbecue.

MISO
Found in the refrigerated food section of health food stores and Asian supermarkets, miso is usually made from soybeans, although it can also be made from rice, barley, wheat, or chickpeas.

MORI-NU TOFU

This shelf-stable tofu can be found in the Asian section of most grocery stores, but it is sometimes kept with produce. Buy Mori-Nu Lite if possible.

NONDAIRY MILK

Soy milk, rice milk, hemp milk, oat milk, and almond milk are just some of the many kinds of nondairy milk on the market. WestSoy makes a fat-free soy milk, but many other brands make light nondairy milks that have a marginal amount of fat. These milks can be used interchangeably in recipes, so feel free to use any type of milk you enjoy or have on hand.

NUTRITIONAL YEAST

Nutritional yeast is a deactivated yeast, meaning it doesn't make breads rise the way active yeast does. Nutritional yeast is a complete protein, low in fat and sodium, and fortified with vitamin B12. It also gives food a cheesy flavor. It can be found at health food stores and vitamin retailers like GNC and the Vitamin Shoppe. I highly recommend Red Star brand, which can be found in some stores and bought in bulk online.

POULTRY SEASONING

Poultry seasoning is a blend of basil, rosemary, thyme, sage, marjoram, and oregano, but other herbs may be included. Avoid buying powdered poultry spice or chicken spice rubs, which can be salty. Look for a granulated poultry spice or make your own blend using the recipe on page 268.

POWDERED SUGAR

Also called confectioners' sugar, powdered sugar is fine and powderlike. You can make your own by combining one cup of raw sugar with two tablespoons of cornstarch in your food processor and letting the motor run until a fine powder is formed.

PUMPKIN PIE SPICE

This blend of cinnamon, ginger, cloves, and nutmeg gives pumpkin pie and other pumpkin foods that distinct flavor we know and love.

PURE MAPLE SYRUP

Pure maple syrup is a delicious natural, unrefined sweetener. Imitation maple syrups and pancake syrups cannot be substituted without sacrificing taste and quality. Agave nectar

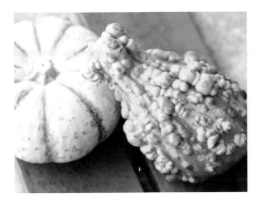

can be substituted for pure maple syrup, but the taste will be different.

PURE PUMPKIN

Pure pumpkin is different from pumpkin pie mix. (Don't use that.) You want canned pure pumpkin or the insides of an actual pumpkin. In a pinch, you can substitute canned sweet potato or potato squash.

QUINOA

Although technically a pseudocereal, quinoa is commonly treated as a grain. It has a nutty flavor and is full of calcium, iron, and magnesium. Quinoa is also a complete protein and cooks quickly, making it a perfect substitute for rice, oatmeal, and other grains when your time is limited. Most U.S. brands of quinoa have been prerinsed, but if your quinoa has a chalky coating,

rinse it several times before cooking or it will taste bitter and soapy. Quinoa bought from the bulk bin should always be rinsed before cooking.

RAW SUGAR

Also called turbinado sugar, raw sugar is a natural, unrefined sugar made from cane juice.

TAMARI

Interchangeable with low-sodium soy sauce in recipes, tamari is similar to low-sodium soy sauce but thicker and usually gluten-free.

TEMPEH

Essentially, tempeh is fermented soybean cakes originating from Indonesia. You can find tempeh at health food stores and in well-stocked supermarkets.

TOFU

There are two distinct types of tofu: tofu that is refrigerated and sitting in water, and tofu (such as Mori-Nu) that is packaged in Tetra Paks and is shelf-stable. Tetra Pak–packaged tofu is very soft and delicate. Refrigerated tofu has a much firmer texture, making it a great replacement for meat. There are several kinds of refrigerated tofu: soft or silken, which is delicate; firm; extra-firm; and super-protein, which is the hardest. The consistency of tofu also changes when it is fried, cooked, baked, or frozen and later thawed.

VEGAN CHOCOLATE CHIPS

Many semisweet chocolate chips are unintentionally vegan. Ghirardelli is my favorite brand.

VEGAN YOGURT

Yogurt made from soy, rice, almond, or coconut milk instead of dairy. If you have a dairy allergy or are vegan, make sure the cultures are not from dairy as well.

VITAL WHEAT GLUTEN

Gluten is the protein found in wheat. It's what gives bread its shape and pizza dough its elasticity. When steamed, baked, boiled, or otherwise cooked, gluten becomes chewy, with a meatlike texture, and is referred to as seitan. Gluten also works as a binding agent, helping hold things like mushroom burgers together. You can find vital wheat gluten in the baking section of health food stores or online.

recipe substitutions

I like to use dried rather than fresh herbs and spices in my recipes because I always have them on hand, they're cheaper, it saves an additional five minutes of prep time, and I dirty fewer dishes. I still love fresh ingredients though, especially those I've grown myself, so here is a handy substitution chart if you'd like to use fresh. I can't guarantee the results will be the same, and you may need to do a little tweaking as you go, but in theory these swaps should work fine.

FRESH » DRIED HERBS

1 tbsp fresh = 1 tsp dried

Note: If I specify fresh herbs in a recipe, dried herbs cannot substitute for them.

ONION » ONION POWDER

1 small onion (⅓ c diced) = 1 tsp onion powder

1 small onion (⅓ c diced) = 1 tbsp onion flakes

GARLIC » GARLIC POWDER

1 clove = ½ tsp minced garlic

1 clove = ¼ tsp garlic powder (granulated)

1 clove = ⅛ tsp garlic powder (flour consistency)

LEMON » LEMON JUICE

1 lemon = 2–3 tbsp lemon juice

1 lemon wedge = ¼–1 tsp lemon juice

Note: Fresh lemon juice is much more potent than store-bought juices. Use fresh whenever possible, adding lemon or lime juice from a bottle to taste.

DRIED BEANS » CANNED BEANS

1¼–1¾ c cooked beans = 15 oz canned beans

SUGAR REPLACEMENT

You can safely reduce sugar by ¼ in any recipe, or use these other sweeteners instead of sugar:

REPLACEMENT FOR 1 CUP OF SUGAR	ADDITIONAL CHANGES
¾ c barley malt syrup	Reduce liquid by ¼
⅔ c date sugar	(no reduction)
1 c fruit syrup	Reduce liquid by ¼
1 c pure maple syrup	Reduce liquid by 3 tbsp, add ¼ tsp baking soda
1 c Sucanat	(no reduction)
1 tsp powdered stevia	(no reduction)

TIP: Take care with substitutions and adaptations. When making a change, ask yourself, "What does the original ingredient do? Does my substitute have the same texture, taste, consistency, color, and feel as the original?" Sometimes changing one thing changes everything.

kitchen prep lingo

I remember my early days in the kitchen. They were filled with questions like "How small is a small onion?" or "What is the difference between mince and chop?" To help cut back on your online searches, I've created this cheat sheet of terms you'll run across in this cookbook.

ALMOST COMBINED/JUST COMBINED
Do not completely combine ingredients. With batter, some flour should still be visible for it to be almost combined. To be just combined, stir it just a little bit more—ingredients should be mixed together and incorporated, but barely. Use as few strokes as possible. (Compare with Blend.)

BEANS
Use canned beans, drained and rinsed, unless the recipe specifically calls for dried beans.

BLEND
Stir to incorporate all ingredients until they are well combined and the mix is homogenous.

CHOP
Cut ingredient into bite-size pieces; uniform cuts are not necessary, and size is relatively unimportant (it's more of a personal preference).

COOKED
A vegetable prepared by steaming, baking, or boiling until fork-tender (seeded and/or skinned prior to cooking if necessary).

CREAM
Beat the ingredients with an electric mixer until they are well combined and have a creamy consistency. This also can be done by hand with a spatula.

CRUMBLE
Break the ingredient apart into smaller pieces. With tofu, break the tofu apart until it resembles ricotta or feta cheese.

FOLD
Gently stir a single ingredient into a mixture, such as muffin batter,

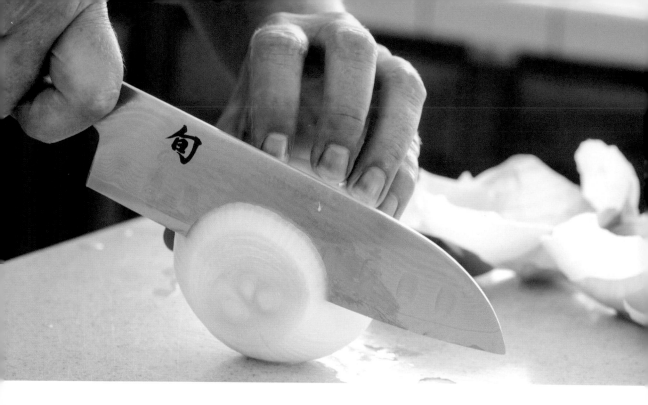

with a spatula or large spoon until just combined.

LINE (WITH WATER OR BROTH)
Add a thin layer of liquid that just barely covers the bottom of the pot or skillet. Start with ¼ cup.

MINCE
Chop ingredients into very small pieces, ⅛ inch or smaller.

ONION
Small onions are the size of a lemon, medium onions are roughly the size of an orange, and large onions are the size of a grapefruit.

SALT AND PEPPER TO TASTE
½ teaspoon of salt and ¼ teaspoon of pepper is usually a good starting point for recipes that serve at least two. Reduce salt if you're using ingredients with sodium, such as canned goods or low-sodium soy sauce. Double as necessary to achieve your preferred taste.

STIR
Use a circular motion, clockwise or counterclockwise, to move or incorporate ingredients.

additional resources

RECOMMENDED READING

The Pleasure Trap: Mastering the Hidden Force that Undermines Health and Happiness by Douglas J. Lisle and Alan Goldhamer; Book Publishing Co. (2006).

Breaking the Food Seduction: The Hidden Reasons Behind Food Cravings—and 7 Steps To End Them Naturally by Neal D. Barnard and Joanne Stepaniak; St. Martin's Griffin; reprint edition (2004).

The End of Overeating: Taking Control of the Insatiable American Appetite by David A. Kessler; Rodale; reprint edition (2010).

Whole: Rethinking the Science of Nutrition by T. Colin Campbell and Howard Jacobson; BenBella Books (2013).

OTHER RECOMMENDED BOOKS

The China Study: The Most Comprehensive Study of Nutrition Ever Conducted and the Startling Implications for Diet, Weight Loss, and Long-term Health by T. Colin Campbell and Thomas M. Campbell II; BenBella Books (2004).

Prevent and Reverse Heart Disease: The Revolutionary, Scientifically Proven, Nutrition-Based Cure by Caldwell B. Esselstyn Jr.; Avery; first edition (2008).

The Engine 2 Diet: The Texas Firefighter's 28-Day Save-Your-Life Plan that Lowers Cholesterol and Burns Away the Pounds by Rip Esselstyn; Grand Central Publishing; first edition (2009).

The Starch Solution: Eat the Foods You Love, Regain Your Health, and Lose the Weight for Good! by John McDougall and Mary McDougall; Rodale; first edition (2012).

Dr. Neal Barnard's Program for Reversing Diabetes: The Scientifically Proven System for Reversing Diabetes without Drugs by Neal D. Barnard; Rodale; first edition (2006).

FILMS

Forks Over Knives (2011)

King Corn (2007)

metric conversions

ABBREVIATION KEY

tsp = teaspoon
tbsp = tablespoon
dsp = dessert spoon

U.S. STANDARD	U.K.	
¼ tsp	¼	tsp (scant)
½ tsp	½	tsp (scant)
¾ tsp	½	tsp (rounded)
1 tsp	¾	tsp (slightly rounded)
1 tbsp	2½	tsp
¼ cup	¼	cup minus 1 dsp
⅓ cup	¼	cup plus 1 tsp
½ cup	⅓	cup plus 2 dsp
⅔ cup	½	cup plus 1 tbsp
¾ cup	½	cup plus 2 tbsp
1 cup	¾	cup plus 2 dsp

index

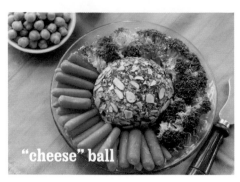

"cheese" ball

C

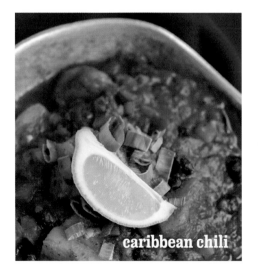

caribbean chili

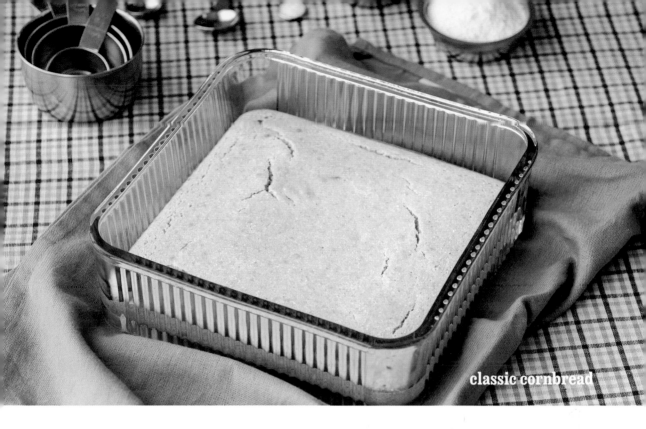

classic cornbread

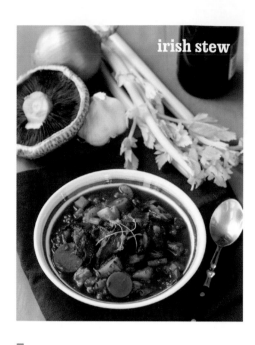

irish stew

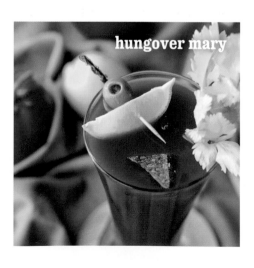

hungover mary

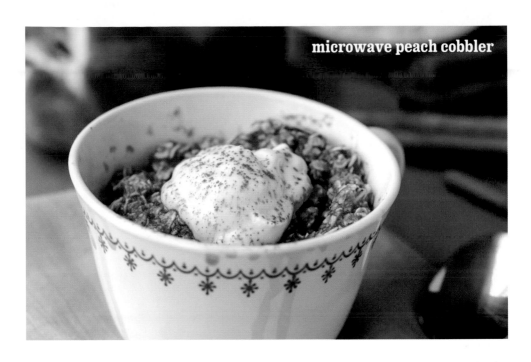

microwave peach cobbler

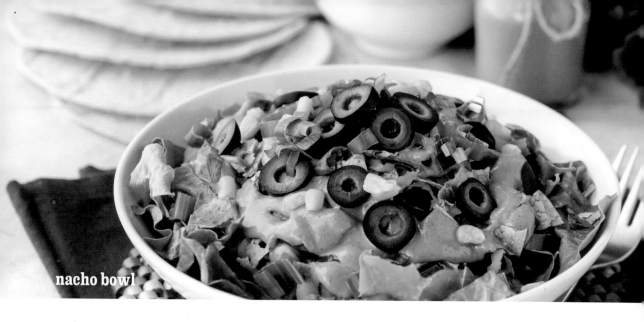

nacho bowl

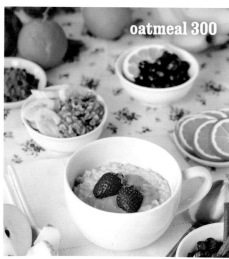

oatmeal 300

P

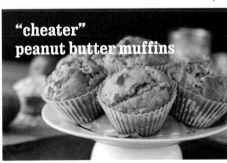

"cheater" peanut butter muffins

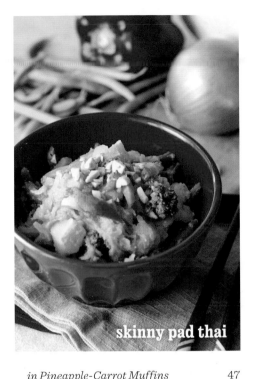

skinny pad thai

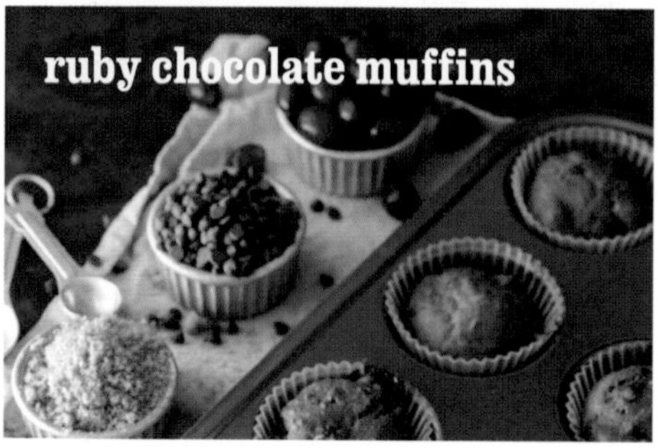

ruby chocolate muffins

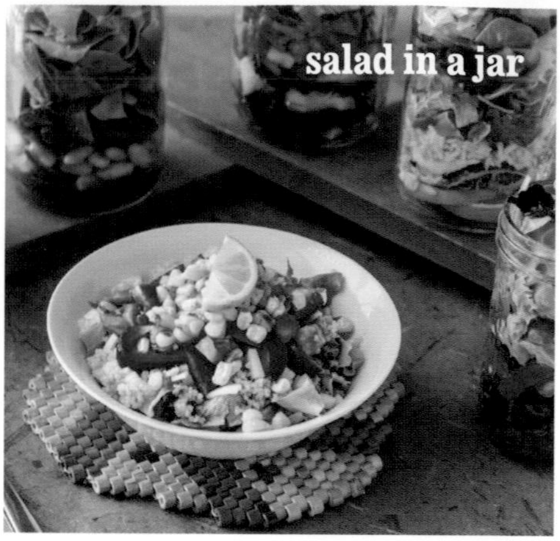

salad in a jar

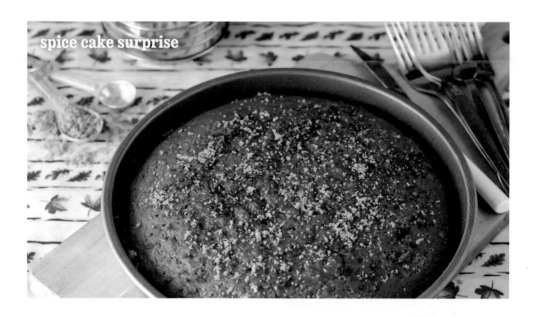

spice cake surprise

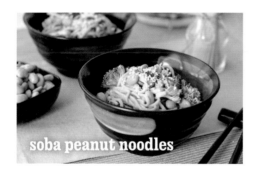

soba peanut noodles

T

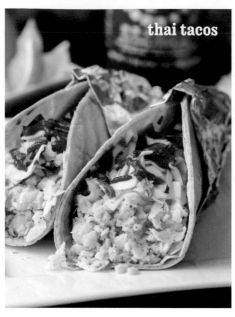

thai tacos

V

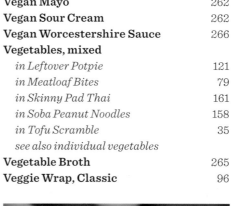

tropical taco salad

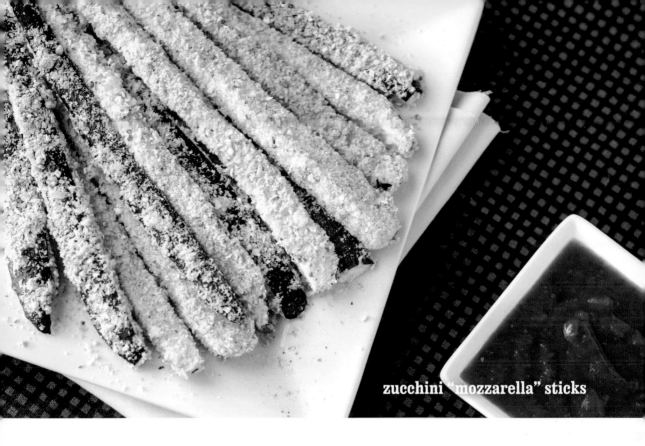

zucchini "mozzarella" sticks

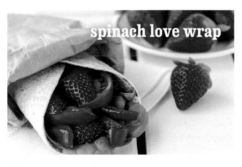

spinach love wrap

acknowledgments

I am thankful every day for the support of my friends, family, and most importantly—my fans (called "Herbies"). I would not have the opportunity to write cookbooks if it weren't for them. Herbies, everything I do, I do for you. Each of you enriches my life and it is my honor to be a part of your journey. Thank you.

I would also like to acknowledge my publisher and the entire BenBella Books team. It takes many hands to make these books happen. I couldn't do it without their talent, dedication, and support.

A special thank-you to my husband, Scott Nixon. I still don't know what I did to deserve such a loving and supportive husband. Let it be known: I could not do what I do without you beside me. Jackie Sobon, thank you for bringing my recipes to life with your beautiful photos; thank you Neely Roberts for your photo contributions here and every week with the meal plans; and thanks also to Natala and Matt Constantine for taking beautiful pictures of me for the cover and the Lean section.

Jon Warren, thank you for cowriting the Lean section with me, and also for showing me how strong I am. I approach life with the attitude of "beast mode" now. You've helped make me my best self and I know I've made you at least a little bit vegan.

My parents, Richard and Lenore Shay, nothing will ever make me as happy as the day you both went plant-based. Also, a special thanks to my father for constantly giving me new ideas for recipes.

Lastly, I am so incredibly thankful for my testers—Dana Strickland, Kim and Stephen Treanor (and girls), Katharina Ikels, Pragati Sawhney Coder, Becky Soubeyrand, Jared Bigman, Nita Ruggiero, Matthew Dempsey, Lisa Canada and Family, the Savage family, Pam Wertz, MarieRoxanne Veinotte, Shereé Britt, Ashley and Michael Nebel, Gin Stafford, Kait Scalisi, Gayle Pollick, Leslie Conn, Dirk Wethington, Candace Sharp, Kimberly Roy, Meagan Brown, Jane Brunk, Jennifer Kent, Candy Guerra, Jenny Calderon, Suzanne Correnti, and Lisa Yost. My books could not exist without your hard work and dedication.

about the author

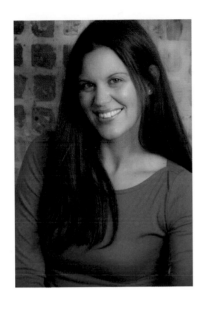

Lindsay S. Nixon is the best-selling author of the Happy Herbivore cookbook series: *The Happy Herbivore Cookbook* (2011), *Everyday Happy Herbivore* (2011), *Happy Herbivore Abroad* (2012), and now *Happy Herbivore Light & Lean*. As of September 2012, Nixon has sold more than 150,000 cookbooks.

Nixon has been featured on the Food Network and *The Dr. Oz Show*, and she has spoken at Google's Pittsburgh office about health, plant-based food, and her success. Her recipes have also been featured in the *New York Times*, *Vegetarian Times* magazine, *Shape* magazine, *Bust*, *Women's Health*, WebMD, and numerous other publications. Nixon's work has also been praised and endorsed by notable leaders in the field of nutrition, including Dr. T. Colin Campbell, Dr. Caldwell B. Esselstyn Jr., Dr. Neal Barnard, Dr. John McDougall, and Dr. Pam Popper.

A rising star in the culinary world, Nixon is recognized for her ability to use everyday ingredients to create healthy, low-fat recipes that taste just as delicious as they are nutritious. For more recipes and information visit happyherbivore.com. You can also try her 7-Day Meal Plans at Getmealplans.com.

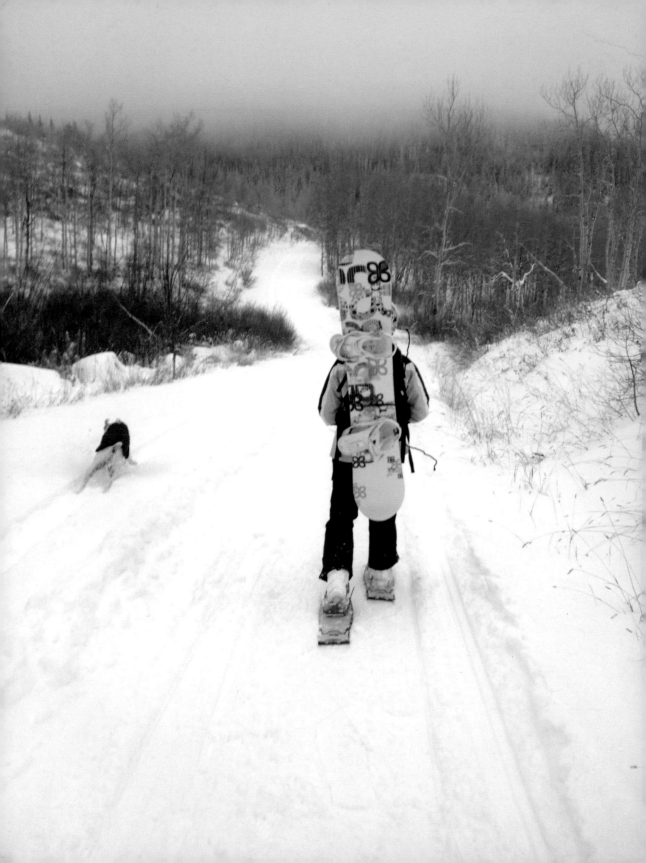